Pilates

STEFANIE RAHN I CHRISTIAN LUTZ

PILATES

COMPLETE TRAINING FOR A SUPPLE BODY

MEYER & MEYER SPORT

British Library Cataloguing in Publication Data
A catalogue library for this book is available from the British Library

Pilates
Maidenhead: Meyer & Meyer Sport (UK) Ltd., 2020
ISBN: 978-1-78255-186-7

Aachen, Auckland, Beirut, Cairo, Cape Town, Dubai, Hägendorf, Hong Kong, Indianapolis, Maidenhead, Manila, New Delhi, Singapore, Sydney, Tehran, Vienna

 Member of the World Sport Publishers' Association (WSPA), www.w-s-p-a.org

Printed by Print Consult, GmbH, Munich, Germany

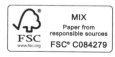

ISBN: 978-1-78255-186-7
Email: info@m-m-sports.com
www.thesportspublisher.com

CONTENTS

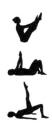

ACKNOWLEDGMENTS

With this book we have fulfilled a long-time dream: to pool our joint knowledge and make the Pilates concept accessible to lots of people.

Our plan met with lots of approval during our research and project implementation. Our collegial exchange and joint work made us realize how valuable and rewarding it is to work as a team, and we would like to express our gratitude for all the support we received.

We are particularly grateful to Meyer & Meyer Sport for their faith in us and for entrusting us with this project; the Artzt firm for making these outstanding photos possible and for allowing us the use of their training equipment; and Winshape for their products.

We would also like to thank the German Pilates Association as well as the German Gymnastics Association for their support.

Stefanie Rahn
Christian Lutz

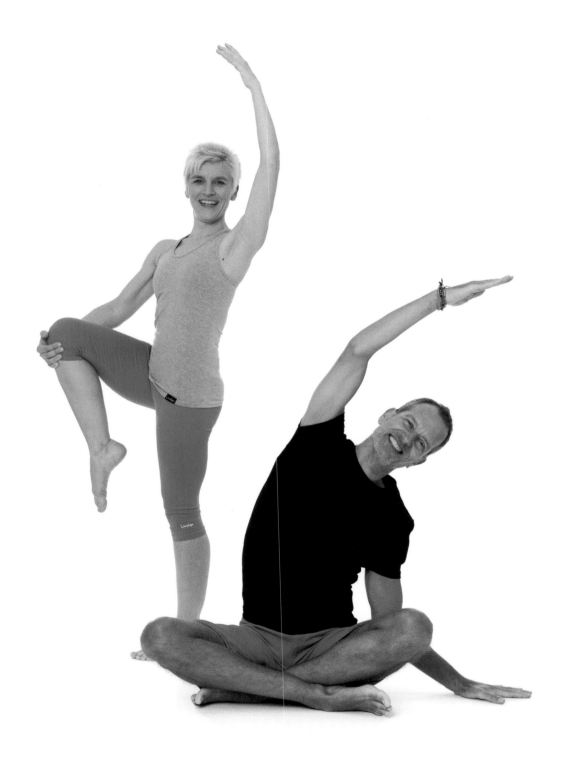

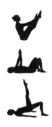

1   PROLOGUE

My job as a sport scientist and osteopath and my career as a performance athlete have taught me the importance of working with great instructors and healthcare professionals. And I often realized that it is not just our physical condition that is pivotal. The mental component—the healthy mind in a healthy body—is just as important. During a competition, the course for victory or defeat is set way ahead of time. When I look at the life and work of Joseph Pilates, I understand very well why his method is still practiced today, and why his philosophy is prevalent around the world. Many of his ideas were ahead of their time and are more topical now than ever. I can see many similarities between his and my mindset: for instance, the desire to help people with our work. Sensible physical and mental work contributes significantly to a better life and greater productivity. In trying to work sensibly, I am—as was Pilates—a pragmatist and allow myself to be inspired by my daily work. Engaging with function and structure and dealing with systems instead of individual parts are additional commonalities. Although I am not explicitly familiar with every facet of his work, I can say that I am very impressed with his ideas, his attitude, and his unerring conviction that exercise heals. So when asked to write a prologue for this book, I immediately accepted. Like Stefanie and Christian, I, too, value the tried and tested while being open to the new. You can read this book as an instructor or active student and practice or teach the many classic exercises with enthusiasm as Pilates had intended, and be open to the many big and small variations.

Edo Hemar

In terms of its complexity, variety, and adaptability, the Pilates method is hard to beat. The Pilates instructor must be very competent in order to lead the exercises in detail and with precision, and the student is asked to follow these instructions and translate them into physical movement. Countless Pilates books have been written, DVDs have been produced, and YouTube and Facebook are rife with Pilates athletes demonstrating their skills. With this book, Stefanie and Christian have managed beautifully to highlight the essence of the Pilates method, to communicate the movements concisely, and to place the focus on precision of movement. The emphasis is placed on the three most important Pilates principles—breathing, centering, and alignment—allowing the student to focus on the substance. The excellent photos in this book are a feast for the eyes and allow even beginners to easily replicate the gymnastic exercises. The mastery of effectively teaching this intelligent exercise method is in meeting the participant at his current level and to further his abilities without overwhelming him. With this book, Stefanie and Christian don't just demonstrate their core competency as outstanding instructors, teachers, and trainers. Their joy and passion reach participants at every single PILATES Bodymotion workshop they teach. Stefanie enchants and touches everyone with her bubbly, funny, and smart personality. And Christian, with his approachable and sensitive personality, inspires confidence in one's own abilities. Paired with a highly professional teaching style and broad expertise, the spark of the passion for this method leaps to the participants and carries everyone along on the Pilates journey that will ideally last a lifetime. It is our great pleasure and gain to have these two special people on our training-instructor team!

Britta Brechtefeld and Ute Weiler

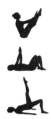

2   MOTIVATION AND INTRODUCTION

The idea to write a Pilates book stemmed from our long-time activity as Pilates students, instructors, and training instructors. Our bodies have spent countless hours in our own training sessions, classes, and workshops. We have an ongoing exchange with colleagues from a variety of orientations, whose questions and suggestions both enrich us and inspire us to reevaluate our own actions. We are united by our fascination with the Pilates method, the Pilates philosophy, and their unbelievable bandwidth.

With this book, we hope to create a broad base to bring this method anywhere we believe it belongs: every living room, every gym or athletic field, every medical practice or rehab facility, every fitness studio or health center. Anywhere people wish to learn sensible exercise. Pilates—with its training principles, as an independent form of exercise, a functional supplement to sport-specific training methods, and an effective physical therapy method—simply belongs.

The outside perception of Pilates is still that of a mere gymnastics program practiced on a mat by women. In fact, Pilates is a functional exercise program that uses various implements and offers countless possibilities.

This book will provide you with the essential basic knowledge under consideration of current scientific findings and research results. Every theoretical digression is made tangible and accessible via practical exercises and can be immediately implemented. The body of the book includes target group-specific exercise programs with and without small implements. In addition to the exercise description we have included tips and suggestions for instructors and students. It is our wish to support instructors and participants in integrating the Pilates method into their training programs and to help Pilates occupy its proper place in the world of sports and healthcare.

2.1   WHAT IS PILATES?

Pilates is a well thought-out, intelligent, and extensive exercise concept. It promotes concentration ability, strength, and flexibility, and is alterable and adaptable with respect to the student and his exercise goals. The frequently cited exercises that are anchored in the public consciousness, such as "One Hundred," represent only a fraction of the exercise repertoire. These frequently cited exercises are much like an iceberg of which only the tip is visible. Some consider the Pilates method a classic that is firmly entrenched in the world of exercise and healthcare, while others still consider it a dark horse. And as extensive and detailed knowledge about the life and work of Joseph Pilates, his method, his milieu, his way of working and his equipment is, as little does the broader public know about it so far. And that's in spite of the fact that over the past 30 years, the name Pilates has appeared in countless magazines, books, articles, broadcasts, and programs. Even its entry into physical therapy and rehabilitation, high-performance sports, and, of course, the exercise programs of prominent performers has not resulted in a breakthrough. Joseph Hubertus Pilates was actually way ahead of his time. His exercise program is well thought out all the way through and represents the complete coordination of body and mind (Pilates & Miller, 2003, pg. 9).

He says about his method, which he called contrology:

Contrology develops the body uniformly, corrects wrong posture, restores physical vitality, invigorates the mind, and elevates the spirit. In childhood, with rare exceptions, we all enjoy the benefits of natural and normal physical development. However, as we mature, we find ourselves living in bodies not always complimentary to our ego. Our bodies are slumped, our shoulders are stooped, our eyes are hollow, our muscles are flabby, and our vitality extremely lowered, if not vanished. This is but the natural result of not having uniformly developed all the muscles of our spine, trunk, arms, and legs in the course of pursuing our daily labors and office activities. (Pilates & Miller, 2003, pg. 9).

Contrology facilitates the body's uniform development, corrects poor posture, restores physical vitality, and invigorates mind and soul. During childhood we tend to benefit from a natural and normal physical development. But as we get older we find ourselves in bodies that don't always seem flattering. Our bodies have caved in, our shoulders slump, our eyes sink deep into their sockets, our muscles are slack, and our vitality is very low, if not gone completely. It is the sad consequence of neglecting our trunk, arm, and leg muscles due to our daily workload (Übers. S. Rahn).

Joseph Pilates wrote those words in 1945. More than 70 years have passed since then, but we still struggle with the same problems. One more reason to continue to spread the Pilates concept.

2.2   JOSEPH H. PILATES AND HISTORY

Joe Pilates was born Joseph Hubertus Pilates on December 9, 1883, in Mönchengladbach, Germany. It was a time of rapid industrialization during which Germany developed from an agrarian society into an industrial state. This time period was characterized by economic fluctuations during which heyday and depression alternated. Hard physical work for women and children was still the order of the day, and living and working conditions for laborers were bad. That was also the case in the Pilates household. His mother Helena Pilates, nee Hahn, (1860-1901), worked in a factory, and his father Heinrich Friedrich (Fritz) Pilates (1859-1922) was an assistant locksmith.

At that time, the infant and maternal mortality rate dropped significantly due to improved hygiene, medical advancements, and better nutrition, and the population of the German Empire sharply increased. Particularly in the urban centers of large cities, the population pressure intensified, and an overseas emigration wave during the 1880s and 1890s was followed by the biggest domestic migratory movement in German history. By the time he was 16 years old, the life of Joseph Pilates was also shaped by constant moves.

⚱ PILATES

He had what it took to pursue a respectable career as a beer brewer, but his fascination with and love of exercise and the development of a strong and supple body caused him to repeatedly leave his job to pursue his passion.

From the time he was young, Joseph Pilates observed the seemingly effortless yet powerful movements of animals, and later, with enthusiasm, his daughter's physical development: kicking her legs, stretching, reaching, rolling over, pushing up, and crawling.

He meticulously practiced the complex sequences of gymnastics and boxing. He learned about the muscles responsible for the different motion sequences from an anatomy book, a gift from his mother's physician. He developed a good eye and a high awareness for the movements of the human body, exercised passionately, and developed from a skinny boy into a muscular young man.

The concept of a body culture emerged with natural exercise sequences, and as a result, Pilates turned more to boxing because the motion sequences in gymnastics seemed increasingly unnatural to him. In Eugen Sandow, Elisabeth Mensendiek, and Genevieve Stebbins, he found role models for a movement and exercise culture intended to help people move better, become healthy in mind and body, and maintain their good health for a lifetime. Next to the correct execution of his exercises, letting go and relaxing as well as consciously using the breath were new exercise principles that had previously attracted little interest in the gymnastics and boxing world he was familiar with.

In November 1913, after the death of his wife Maria, Joseph Pilates emigrated to England. The assertion made by other sources that Pilates had already left for England as a boxer in 1912, cannot be verified. However, there is proof he personally registered his wife's death at the civil registry office in November 1913.

Whatever the reason Pilates left Germany and whatever his occupation might have been in England, WW I brought it all to an abrupt halt. Germans, Turks, and Austrians (men between the ages of 17 and 55) were declared foreign aliens and interned. The dreary surroundings, the lack of power over their situation, and the forced inactivity quickly led to a desolate and depressive mood amongst the prisoners.

Joseph Pilates' moment had come. To counter the hopelessness surrounding him, he began to organize activities and exercised his fellow prisoners with a kind of boxing gymnastics to keep them physically and mentally fit.

In the fall of 1915, he was moved to Camp Knockaloe on the Isle of Man, a giant camp with better infrastructure and more opportunity for activities. Here Pilates became part of an up-and-coming boxing culture that not only included athletic aspects, but also became an important social event in everyday prison life.

Pilates began to observe animals again (here cats in particular) and developed a training concept that would both stretch and strengthen the body by consciously performing the exercises in due consideration of specific training principles. (Romana Kryzanowska once defined the Pilates method as a two-way stretch with a strong core.)

Pilates may have gotten the idea to use springs for resistance in his apparatuses in Knockaloe. They were intended to stimulate the tissue's tensile resistance against which students would vigorously stretch.

After the end of WWI, Pilates returned to Germany in March 1919, and in the following years focused more on the sport of boxing. He established his own boxing school and even fought several matches.

But he still continued work on his exercise plan and invented apparatuses to facilitate these exercises. In August 1922, he submitted his first patent application for the foot corrector to the patent office of the German Reich in Berlin. It was approved in May 1923.

Due to the bad economic climate in Germany, Joseph Pilates' younger brother Fritz left Germany for America in 1923.

During the summer of 1923, Pilates found a job as a self-defense instructor for the Hamburg police department. There he learned the Japanese martial art Jiu- Jitsu, which purposefully uses the opponent's hands as resistance during training and specifically integrates breathing into the practice. He promoted good physical hygiene and added the concept of free body culture (nudism) with its dislike of clothing that prevents the rays of the sun from accessing the human body to his method.

In August 1924, Joseph Pilates received the patent for his physical training apparatus—later known as the Universal Reformer—in Hamburg. That same year, Joseph Pilates met the American boxing journalist Nat Fleischer, who was excited about his method and his physical training apparatus, and convinced him to travel to New York for the first time in 1925.

In 1926, Joseph Pilates left Germany for good and moved his residence to New York. During his ocean passage, he met Clara Zeuner (1883-1976), his subsequent life companion and major supporter in bringing his plans to fruition.

With help from Nat Fleischer, Joseph Pilates found a space for his studio at 939 8th Avenue between 55th and 56th Street. There Joseph Pilates worked with his first clients primarily on his physical training apparatus, for which he now also owned a patent in America under the name Gymnastic Apparatus. On his business card, he changed the year of his birth to 1880.

In spite of the global economic crisis, Pilates was able to establish his studio and acquire a good reputation in the world of dance. Working with Ruth St. Denis and Ted Shaw resulted in a regular teaching job at the Summer Camp for Dancers at Jacob's Pillow in the Berkshires starting in 1941.

In the meantime he had published his first book, Your Health, in 1934, which was followed by Return to Life through Contrology in 1945. This book was an invitation to all people to exercise according to his method and improve their lives in the process. It includes 34 exercises that can be done anywhere and requires only one's own body as a training tool.

Later efforts to make his method accessible to the American medical profession and establish it as part of the healthcare system in the United States failed. The extent to which Joseph Pilates was convinced of his method's effectiveness is evident in a letter written in 1961, to the then president of the United States, John F. Kennedy, in which he offers to improve the government's physical fitness program through his concepts.

During the following years, Pilates withdraw more and more from his studio. He reduced his own exercise regimen and largely neglected his body. He became seriously ill in 1965. Pulmonary emphysema caused him severe breathing problems and even made climbing the steps to his studio difficult.

At the end of September 1967, he was hospitalized at Lenox Hill Hospital in New York with severe respiratory distress and died there on October 9, 1967.

2.3 THE STATUS QUO

Although he was born and raised in Germany, it is taking a long time for the Pilates method to become known here and it is spreading very slowly. While the first studios in Great Britain were created as far back as the 1970s, in Germany the first stirrings only took place in the 1980s. The mat exercise program established itself very tentatively in gymnastics, dance, and fitness studios. The first Pilates studios with equipment were set up. Instructor training was still limited to just a few schools. Today, there are approximately 800 Pilates studios in Germany, offering mat exercises and equipment workouts. This translates to approximately 95,000 active members. Sixty-one percent of fitness facilities offer Pilates classes. Pilates is particularly popular in the large German cities like Munich, Cologne, Hamburg, and Berlin. But even in Stuttgart, Frankfurt, Düsseldorf, and Erfurt, relatively many people seek out these class offerings (source: fitogram). However, in rural areas the Pilates spirit has yet to be found. Pilates apparatuses like the Reformer, Trapeze Table, Chair, or Barrel are largely unknown, even among many instructors. And that in spite of the fact that since the founding of the German Pilates Association in 2006, the number of training institutions has increased from 5 to 16. Add to that the many other training opportunities through clubs and associations that have realized that even experienced instructors need more than one weekend to familiarize themselves with the Pilates principles.

We can only guess why Pilates in its entirety is still relatively unknown. One reason may be the lack of a centuries-old history and tradition like that of yoga. The proper training is also long and expensive. Just like the Pilates apparatuses. Their acquisition, use, and amortization are only possible with a well thought-out concept and the appropriate setting. Regardless, we Pilateros and Pilatistas have to take a good look in the mirror. Marketing and networking are not our forte. By the way, that was the case with Joseph Pilates, too, but instead of an excuse it should be an incentive to become more active and publicize the method's many advantages, particularly with respect to other sports. Its reputation as an exercise for women, a stretching program, or relaxation training, still precedes the method. In fact the application of the Pilates principles makes Pilates unique. They invigorate every exercise and make it a special, individual, and target-oriented experience.

2.4   WHO SHOULD PRACTICE PILATES?

Anyone can do Pilates, from the rehab patient to the performance athlete, from the adolescent to the senior citizen. Joseph Pilates developed an exercise method that enables anyone, regardless of age, gender, and fitness level, to master life's tasks with joy and dedication. What matters is the motivation or the goal an interested party brings to the table. Some just want to unwind for an hour each week or be around other people. Others focus on the physiological aspects. People who work want some balance during their lunch break or after work, athletes want to supplement and optimize their training. In cases of injury or illness—like, for instance, a torn ACL, joint replacements, or arthritis—Pilates is the ideal exercise (in consultation and collaboration with the treating physician or therapist, of course) for a quick recovery and to regain lost strength, mobility, stability, and control. While a physical therapist makes sure that the injured body region receives the necessary care, we as instructors can support the rest of the body to reverse compensation and adaptation patterns and restore the desired function. Next to the positive effects on physical health, the method also promotes and helps maintain mental health. The results of studies done with people suffering from depression have verified the positive effects of regular Pilates training (Opitz, 2013).

Participants are motivated by different things that often aren't very well defined. That makes it difficult for us instructors to put together the ideal program. It is a good idea to clarify beforehand what happens in a Pilates class and what Pilates can accomplish, because Pilates is not a universal remedy and does have its limitations. For overweight people, Pilates is an excellent exercise program that helps increase general well-being, body awareness, and an upright posture. But anyone expecting the pounds to melt away will be disappointed. Pilates is also not suited for cardiovascular training, nor does it work as exercise on the side with the television on or while chatting with the neighbor. During their exercise units, our participants must be ready for new physical experiences and bring with them a certain amount of eagerness and diligence (Joseph Pilates recommended 3 times a week). Then Pilates will take full effect resulting in "mens sana in corpore sano."

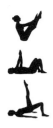

3 TRAINING PRINCIPLES

3.1 PILATES IS A PRINCIPLE-BASED PRACTICE

Joseph H. Pilates based his exercise on a very distinctive philosophy. The traditional Pilates principles subsequently developed from these seminal ideas and considerations. It is less about mindlessly working through a specific exercise sequence, and more about performing the movements in a way that creates the balance between body and mind Joseph Pilates intended (Pilates, 1934). The principles also give structure to the exercise and serve as a kind of guideline the student can always go back to. The instructor uses them as a basis to prepare, compile, and properly teach the exercises. The following principles were listed by Friedman and Eisen in 1980, in their book The Pilates Method of Physical and Mental Conditioning (Friedman, Eisen, 1980, pg. 5), and have been used as the Pilates principles ever since:

- Concentration
- Centering
- Control
- Breathing
- Precision
- Flow

Over the course of the past decades, these principles have been interpreted in different ways, and have been supplemented or increasingly refined. For this book, we decided to make a choice and add the alignment principle to the list. Anyone who practices Pilates will quickly notice that practicing according to and with this valuable principle will result in better quality of execution and, as Joseph Pilates envisioned, the uniform development of the body, correction of poor posture, and restoration of physical vitality (Pilates & Miller, 2000-2005, pg. 9).

3.1.1   BREATHING

BREATHING MAKES A DIFFERENCE

Breathing is certainly the principle that is most different from other types of exercise and gymnastics. It is the breath that makes the exercises special, the thing that makes Pilates what it is, and allows the complete execution of the exercises with respect to strength, flexibility, and relaxation. Moreover, the breath accompanies each exercise, dictates its rhythm and tempo, and is in itself an exercise. The better the breathing technique, the better the execution of the exercise. Regardless of physical limitations and injuries, exercises based on the breathing principle can be performed anywhere, anytime. After all, breathing is the first and last thing a human being does. We can live without food or water for a while, but without breathing life ends within minutes. The breath is the direct link between the inner world and the outer world, and it signals any change in our physical and mental state. Taking belly breaths has a calming effect, while breathing into the upper chest area will cause a sense of panic. Thus, being able to control the tempo, intensity, and direction of one's breath can also mean being able to more consciously direct and control our emotions, moods, and feelings.

The breath may be the most important key to concentration and relaxation. Just think of meditation and relaxation techniques during which the use of conscious, slow breaths lowers the heart rate and blood pressure. This cannot be done by sheer will, only with the breath as a bridge (Laarz, D., 2017, pg. 42). It is also the critical factor in strength and stability. We can hear this in the explosive exhalations of a tennis player during a powerful serve, or during blows and kicks in martial arts.

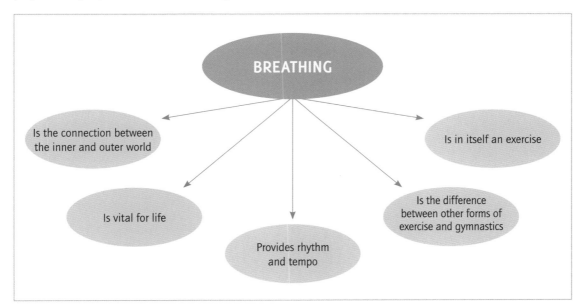

Figure 1

HOW DOES BREATHING WORK?

The diaphragm is the largest respiratory muscle. It is a dome-like structure located in the ribcage between the lower part of the sternum, the lower ribs down to the lumbar vertebrae, and thus separates the belly and the chest. During inhalation the diaphragm works concentrically, flattens, drops, and pushes the abdominal organs down. The chest area enlarges three-dimensionally and the lungs fill with air. The deep abdominal muscle and the pelvic floor relax and lengthen eccentrically to resist the pressure in the abdomen. The opposite pattern takes place during exhalation. The diaphragm returns to its dome shape, the ribs can relax, the abdominal organs return to their previous position. The deep abdominal or thoracic breaths alone allow the organs to experience a regular massage. The ribcage and the thoracic spine are gently moved in all directions. During Pilates, inhalation occurs preferably through the nose, exhalation takes place through the slightly open mouth and is a little throaty, which keeps the jaw loose and relaxed and moderates the pressure in the abdomen. Exaggerated exhalation or loud noises are unnecessary. Instead it is suggested to exhale like a sigh rather than blowing the air out.

A good breathing technique has even more benefits: Due to its position at the inside of the lumbar spine, the diaphragm is able to affect the function of the psoas muscle. The diaphragm spans the fibers of the psoas like a bow and is therefore also able to constrict it when it is taut (see Bohlander, Geweniger, 2011). A flexible diaphragm is essential to an efficient and functioning psoas. Here respiration is directly linked to an upright gait. And due to the diaphragm's functional and fascial connection to the deep abdominal muscle and the pelvic floor, respiration is closely linked to the centering principle. Paying sufficient attention to breathing, particularly when first practicing Pilates, is therefore beneficial in more ways than one, even if it is often confusing to know when one should ideally inhale or exhale during an exercise. The more confident breathing becomes, the easier and self-evident is its use.

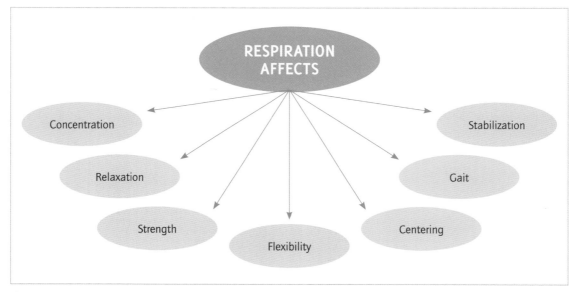

Figure 2

When choosing the breathing exercises, we let ourselves be guided by Eve Gentry. She was an actual student of Joseph Pilates and has further refined his technique because she realized that her students benefitted more from exhaling instead of inhaling upon exertion. It is a frequently seen ground rule. Advanced participants are certainly able to also inhale upon exertion and should practice doing so, particularly since inhalation supports movements in extension. But the exercises in this book are also intended for beginners and amateurs, meaning the people who come to our classes and generally do so only once a week. We therefore deviate from the breathing patterns Joseph Pilates mentioned in his notes.

When describing the exercises, we differentiate between the direction and region in which the breath can flow, and the goal of the exercise, from belly breathing, which is similar to resting respiration, to thoracic breathing, which mobilizes the ribcage and the thoracic spine, all the way to typical Pilates breathing, a functional way of breathing used for all exercises that require strength.

BELLY BREATHING

Goal: Neutral breathing for relaxation.

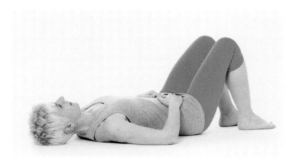

Starting position: Neutral supine position with knees bent and feet planted; legs are parallel and hip-width apart; hands rest on the belly.

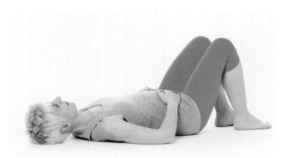

Execution: Inhale through the nose and purposefully direct the breath towards the pelvis, low back, and into the belly. The low back expands; the belly rises and lifts the hands with it.

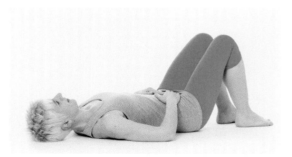

Next, exhale through the slightly open mouth and notice the belly dropping beneath your hands; imagine the abdominal wall resting against the rear of the low back.

TIP:

Place an object (e.g., a light shoe) on your belly to emphasize the activation and receive immediate feedback by seeing the object move up and down.

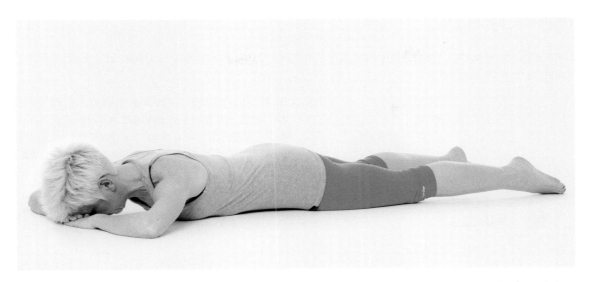

Variation: Belly breathing in a prone position. Here the belly can relax and bulge into the floor, and then lift off the floor and rest against the rear of the low back during exhalation.

THORACIC BREATHING

Goal: Mobilizing the ribcage and thoracic spine and expanding the breathing space on a sagittal plane, meaning forward and back.

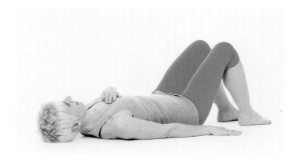

Starting position: Neutral supine position; knees are bent and feet are planted; legs are open hip-width apart; one arm rests alongside the body, the other hand rests on the upper part of the sternum.

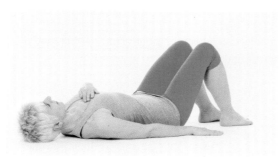

Execution: Purposefully direct the inhalation underneath the upper part of the sternum so the sternum lifts the hand slightly. The collarbones pull sideways, widening the shoulder girdle.

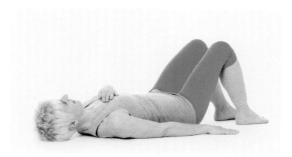

As you exhale, feel the sternum relax; the hand drops and the space between the shoulder blades widens.

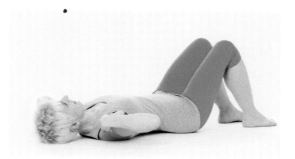

Variation 1: Rest the hands on top of the shoulders; elbows are open to the sides.

As you inhale, gently press the elbows into the floor so the collarbones pull sideways and the thoracic spine stretches slightly.

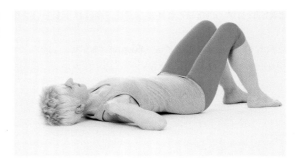

As you exhale, bring the elbows together in front of the body, the shoulder blades widen and the thoracic spine relaxes; the sternum drops between the shoulder blades.

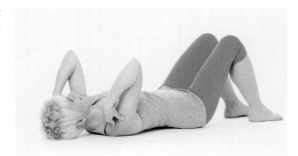

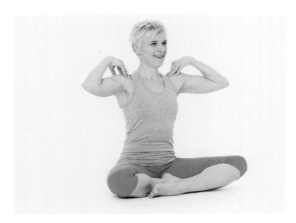

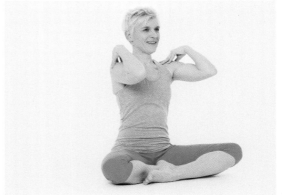

Variation 2: Do variation 1 in a seated position.

BREATHING INTO ONE LUNG WITH ROTATION

Goal: Mobilizing the ribcage and thoracic spine on a horizontal plane. Inhaling into one lung generally results in more mobility and greater range of motion.

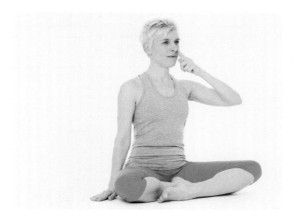

Starting position: Sit in an upright position (on the floor or on a stool); arms are relaxed at your sides. Cover your left nostril with your pinkie.

Preparation: Allow the inhaled breath to flow through the left nostril into the left lung. Repeat several times and then switch sides.

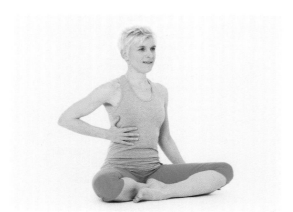

Execution: Place the right hand against the right costal arches for support.

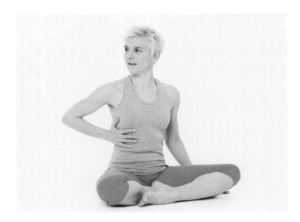

As you exhale, use your right hand to gently push the ribs back into starting position.

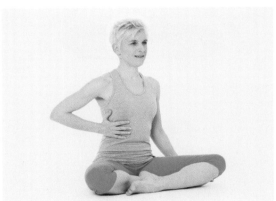

Variation: Some participants respond better to the mental image of the costal arches pulling, while others prefer to imagine the pushing. Purposefully send your inhalation into the right lung as you rotate the spine to the left. The right costal arches push against your right hand, increasing rotation of the ribcage. Reverse the exercise. Purposefully send your inhalation into the left lung as the spine rotates to the right as though the left costal arches were pulling the ribcage into the rotation.

As you exhale, return to the starting position. Continue to alternate sides.

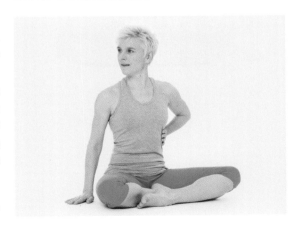

BREATHING INTO ONE LUNG WITH LATERAL FLEXION

Goal: Mobilizing the ribcage and thoracic spine on the frontal plane. Inhaling and exhaling while focusing on just one lung increases lateral flexion and supports erection of the trunk upon return.

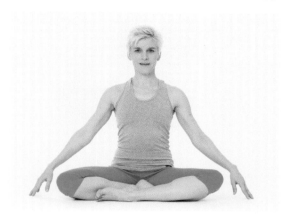

Starting position: Sit in an upright position (on the floor or on a stool); arms are relaxed at your sides.

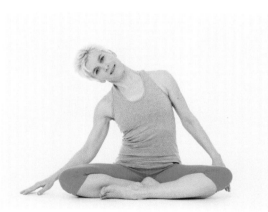

Execution: Send your inhaled breath underneath the left costal arches as you bend the spine to the right (lateral flexion) as though the left costal arches were being pushed up from the inside. The crown of the head reaches sideways into space. Keep looking straight ahead.

Now exhale via only the left lung while moving the left costal arches back into the upright starting position as though the left ribs were pulling the ribcage back in place.

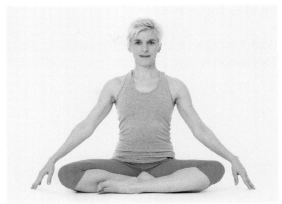

Variation: You can intensify the exercise by extending the left arm up and over. Fingertips reach into space; the left shoulder remains down and the left shoulder blade rests against the ribcage.

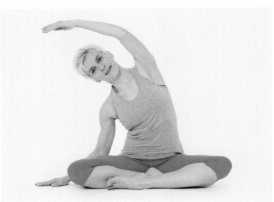

PILATES BREATHING

Goal: Functional breathing while exercising. The air flows into the ribcage and not into the belly so the abdominal muscles can maintain their stabilizing function.

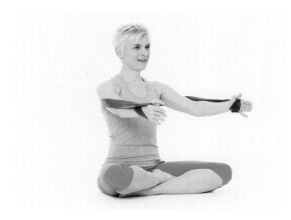

Starting position: Sit in an upright position (on the floor or on a stool); the elastic band is stretched around the back and along the arms; hold the ends in your hands. (See chapter 5.12.3 for optimal wrapping without cutting in.)

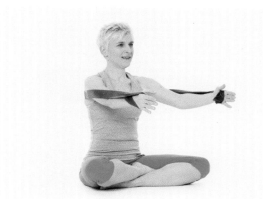

Execution: Purposefully send the inhaled breath under the band, into the back of the ribcage, the back of the lungs. At the same time the arms push the band forward. The ribcage widens primarily to the back and sides. Sit up tall.

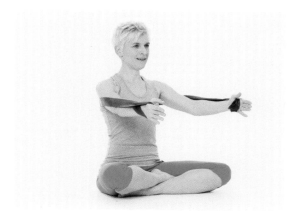

As you exhale, maintain the upright posture and slightly ease up on the tension.

3.1.2 CENTERING

In the Pilates method, initiating movement from a strong and stable core means centering. Every motion impulse is initiated with the proximal (close to the core) activation of the deep trunk muscles. In this context, Joseph Plates himself talked about the girdle of strength, Romana Kryzanowska talked about the power house, and both were referring to the muscles between the ribcage and the pelvis that are responsible for stabilizing the center of the body. When taking a closer look at the anatomy of the trunk, we can see the need for active muscular stabilization.

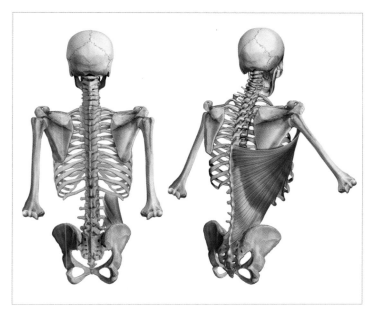

Figure 3: Osseous structure of the trunk with pelvis, ribcage, and spine

With respect to stability, the trunk can be divided into three sections. In the lower section, we have the osseous and very sturdy pelvic ring that protects the pelvic organs and is responsible for the transmission of force between the trunk and the lower extremities. In the upper area, we can see the ribcage, which consists of vertebrae, ribs, sternum, and cartilage, and the pelvis is protective armor (for our vital organs, the heart and lungs) but allows more movement in order to meet respiratory demands. The in-between section, the lumbar spine, does not possess an osseous structure. It needs active muscular stabilization.

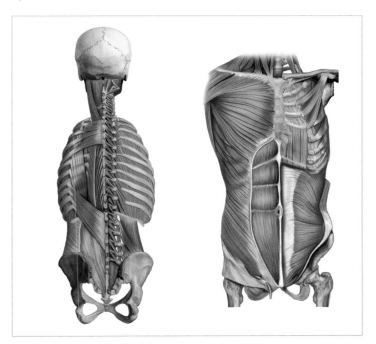

Figure 4: Muscles of the trunk with muscular corset to stabilize the lumbar spine

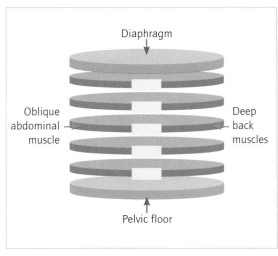

Diaphragm

Oblique abdominal muscle

Deep back muscles

Pelvic floor

Figure 5: Power cylinder

To explain the stabilizing function, we often resort to topographical anatomy, meaning we look at which muscles are located in the area that needs to be stabilized and explore how they work. In the case of the trunk, we can speak of an internal core-control unit, a power cylinder. It is the key to efficient and flowing movement. This power cylinder consists of the pelvic floor at the bottom, the diaphragm at the top, and the abdominal and back muscles as the walls. The coordinated activation of these muscles generates the stability specific to a movement task.

Instructions like, for instance, "Expand the abdominal wall in depth and width like a drumhead" or "Allow the ribs to flow to the pelvis with the exhaled breath," support this activation.

However, in addition to the back and abdominal muscles, there are also other structures in the body that play an important role in stabilizing and controlling the low back. Here we use a different approach to manage movement tasks; it is called functional anatomy. In doing so, we look at functional movement and supporting chains whose parts don't have to be located exclusively in the areas to be stabilized or moved but contribute to accomplishing the movement task. New findings from research on the properties and function of the fasciae (connective tissue) strongly suggests that in addition to the musculature, connective tissue structures also contribute to core stability and control. The model of the deep frontal lines by American Rolfer Thomas Myers shows that stretching the body from the soles of the feet to the crown of the head activates periarticular structures that contribute to the proximal stability of the low back. Moreover, superficial functional lines also help to stabilize and control the core. They are an important part of every functional movement and are used in Pilates exercises. We are talking about functional connectivity between arms, legs, and trunk muscles during stretching, bending, lateral flexion, and rotating movements, but also during supporting functions. The decisive factor for the successful integration of the extremities into the respective functional line is the stable trunk. Of interest in this context are, for example, the works of Kurt Tittel, Leopold Busquet, Paul Chauffour, and the previously mentioned Thomas Myers.

For the practical application in this book, the information given above means:

- We always look at the individual as a whole, his posture as well as his movements.

- Every muscular activity affects neighboring and distant structures.

- We have access to more and more global resources to stabilize our body and to functionally implement movement tasks in the best possible way.

- Moderate activation of various structures of a functional line can be more effective than vigorous activation of an individual structure.

Furthermore we can supplement our mental image of trunk stability with the tensegrity model. This model of the body is based on Buckminster Fuller's architectonic model. Tensegrity (tension = stress, integrity = cohesion) refers to models made of elastic tensile modules and rigid compressive modules. The system's mode of operation is facilitated by the array of the compressive modules that float within the grid of the tensile module. The compressive modules never touch and facilitate the even transfer to the elastic system of external forces that affect the overall system. The system always reacts as a whole to external loads and returns as quickly as possible to its original shape. When overloaded, the system always fails at its weakest point and not inevitably at the point where the load is applied. Tensegrity models are not subject to gravity. We can see many parallels when looking at the human body. While the human body is subject to the effects of gravity, it nevertheless maintains its shape regardless of its position in space. The system that holds our body together and gives it its shape via tension and compression consists of bones and fascial tissue. Every deformation in terms of movement or a change in posture produces a load on the entire system. When we are able to maintain tension in the tensile elements, choosing a load that does not exceed maximal tensile force anywhere in the system, and the tensile elements (i.e., the bones at the joints) do not touch and immediately transfer the pressure, our system remains healthy and in good working order. With regard to our exercises, this means the following:

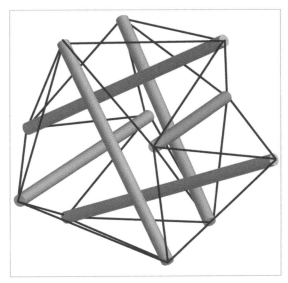

Figure 6: Tensegrity model

- Before we move, our body builds up tension in all directions. ("Imagine your entire body is covered by an elastic bodysuit. Stretch this suit in all directions before you start to move.")

- We never create compression when we move, meaning, for instance, when we do a side bend even the side we bend to maintains length (traction). ("As you move, maintain tension on all sides of your whole-body suit.")

- Wherever bones come together and touch, force is no longer distributed to the total system but rather in just one place. This results in load peaks that can have a negative effect on the overall system.

- Uncontrolled or excessive swinging or pulsing can cause the maximum acceptable tension to be exceeded. Remember that the overall system is only as strong as its weakest component. Possible consequences may be soft tissue injuries (damage) that can negatively affect the overall system.

⚕ PILATES

Thus overloading results in stress to the overall system all the way to discomfort or injuries. With respect to centering, this means that in order to protect the low back, we must also work on the adjacent regions to ensure equal distribution of loads throughout the entire body.

The following are a few examples for practicing with topographical and functional centering.

Topographical:

- Integrate the ribs.

- Allow the ribs to drop towards the pelvis.

- Pull the navel towards the spine.

- The abdominal wall gets deep, wide, and flat.

- Pull the sit bones together.

- Move the pubic symphysis towards the tailbone.

Functionally:

- Create body tension from the soles of the feet to the crown of the head while lying on the back, side, or stomach, or while standing.

- Create body tension from the sit bones to the crown of the head while seated or on all fours.

- Create length and width with the axes of the body.

- Imagine stretching an elastic whole-body suit evenly in all directions.

- Form closed and half-closed force chains by actively working against resistance with your extremities.

- In general, use contact pressure against the floor or a wall to better activate your core (pay attention to neutral alignment).

- Bending the arms and legs and internally rotating the shoulders and hips can aid trunk flexion.

- Extending the arms and legs and externally rotating the shoulders and hips can aid trunk extension.

A FEW PRACTICE EXAMPLES

DIRECTLY TARGETING THE CORE

STERNUM DROP TO ACTIVATE THE UPPER ABDOMINAL MUSCLES

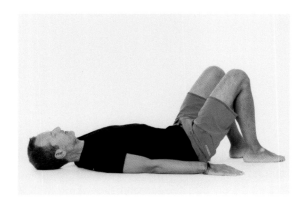

Starting position: Neutral supine position with knees bent; feet are propped in extension of the sit bones.

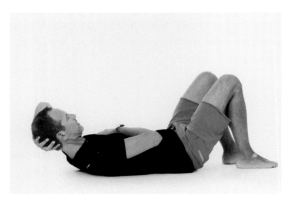

Execution: Place your right hand on your sternum and cradle the back of your head in your left hand. Now activate your abdominal muscles by gently lengthening the cervical spine with the left hand and lifting the head a couple inches off the floor. Still exhaling, roll the chin towards the sternum while simultaneously spreading the sternum towards the pelvis with the right hand and lifting the upper body to the points of the shoulder blades. As you inhale, roll back down to the starting position. Repeat this exercise 5-8x.

Goal: Conscious engagement of the upper abdominal muscles; improved stability and abdominal strength in a neutral supine position; improved awareness of good head alignment.

What to keep in mind: Roll up high enough so you are supported by your abdominal muscles and not your neck muscles. Allow the sternum to drop between the shoulder blades for more axial length and less stress on the nape. Maintain a neutral pelvic position during the entire movement. The abdominal wall remains low, wide, and flat. Don't arch your back!

TIPS FOR PROS

For better awareness of the neutral position, place a small pillow under your lumbar spine. Alternate hands to avoid working one-sided.

LOW ABS TO ACTIVATE DEEP ABDOMINAL MUSCLES AND LOWER ABDOMINAL MUSCLES

Goal: Consciously engaging the deep abdominal muscles (transverse abdominals); improved stability and abdominal strength in a neutral supine position; isolated leg movements.

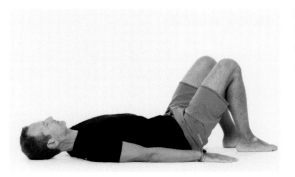

Starting position: Neutral supine position with knees bent; feet are planted in extension of the sit bones; arms are extended alongside the body palms down.

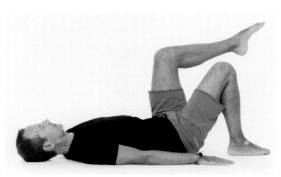

Execution: As you exhale, activate your abdominal muscles and lift the left leg. Allow the left thigh to sink deeply into the hip and slide through it. It should feel like the knee is falling towards the upper body. As you inhale, return the left foot to starting position. Work effortlessly and lightly. Repeat the exercise 3-5x per leg.

Variation: Practice internal and external rotation. For a more challenging exercise, practice with the feet farther away from the pelvis. To add more intensity, lift the legs one after another or at the same time.

What to keep in mind: Maintain a neutral pelvic position during the entire exercise. The abdominal wall remains low, wide, and flat. Don't arch your back!

TIPS FOR PROS

Rest your head on a pillow for better alignment of the head and cervical spine. For better awareness of the neutral position, place a small pillow under the lumbar spine. Keep the calves relaxed to be more aware of the activity of the deep hip flexors.

INDIRECTLY TARGETING THE CORE VIA MYOFASCIAL CHAINS

AXIAL TENSION WHILE STANDING
ACTIVATION OF DEEP FRONTAL LINE AS PER T. MYERS

Goal: Consciously activating the deep and periarticular structures from head to toe; using the transverse abdominals via axial tension; improving awareness of the deep frontal line.

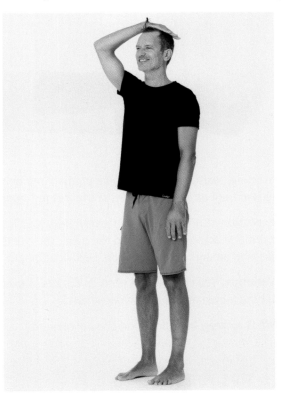

Starting position: Neutral standing position (see orientation and alignment).

Execution: Purposefully and actively press your feet into the floor. Rest one hand on the crown of your head and actively press it into your palm. Feel your body lengthening along its axis and a stabilizing ring forming around your midsection. Hold your breath a few times, then release. Repeat the exercise 1-3x.

Variation: To refine the exercise, activate your medial arches. Feel the strength from the arch of the foot flow up to the knee along the back of the shin. From there it flows along the inside of the thigh to the pelvic floor, from the pelvic floor to the lumbar spine via the deep hip flexors and on up to the diaphragm, along the inside of the ribcage to the first rib, at the front of the cervical spine to the tongue. Gently press the tongue against the roof of the mouth.

What to keep in mind: Good body alignment.

TIPS FOR PROS

Begin by working with the basic exercise description. Gradually add more aspects, provided the participants have the proper awareness. Do not overwhelm your participants with instructions they are not ready for.

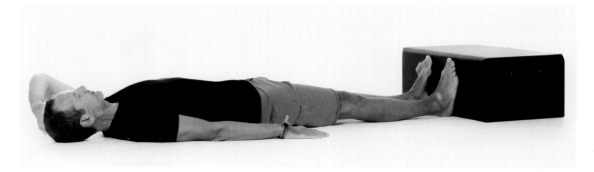
SUPINE POSITION WITH SOLES OF FEET RESTING AGAINST A BOX
FEET PUSHING AGAINST THE BOX ACTIVATES THE DEEP FRONTAL LINE
AS PER T. MYERS

Goal: Consciously activating the deep periarticular structures from head to toe; engaging the transverse obliques via axial tension; improving awareness of deep frontal line.

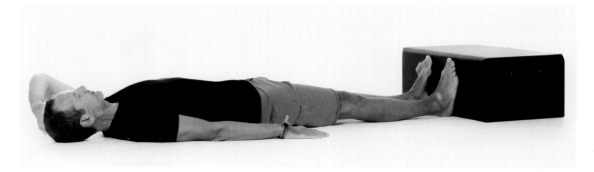

Starting position: Neutral supine position (see orientation and alignment) with extended or slightly bent legs in front of a box; the soles of the feet rest against the box and heels rest on the floor.

Execution: Consciously and actively press your feet against the box. Rest one hand on the crown of the head and actively press it into the palm. Feel yourself lengthening along your axis and a stabilizing ring forming around your midsection. Hold your breath a few times, then release. Repeat the exercise 1-3x.

Variation: You can use this position for lots of exercises in a supine position and generate more support for the movements from the deep muscles.

What to keep in mind: Good body alignment.

TIPS FOR PROS

You can also let the deep frontal line support your movements by integrating the tongue into the movements. Sticking out the tongue supports flexion. Pressing the tongue against the roof of the mouth supports spinal extension. Pressing the tongue against the left or right cheek helps with rotation in the respective direction.

But here, too, the rule is: Do not overwhelm your participants with instructions they are not ready for.

SUPINE POSITION WITH ARMS EXTENDED ABOVE THE STERNUM AND PALMS TOUCHING PRESS THE PALMS TOGETHER TO ACTIVATE THE OBLIQUES

Goal: Consciously activating the oblique muscles of the trunk via the arms.

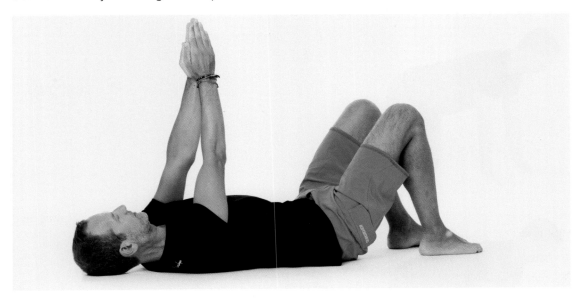

Starting position: Neutral supine position (see alignment) with extended or bent legs; feet are planted hip-width apart parallel to the floor; arms are extended above the lower half of the sternum; palms touch.

Execution: Vigorously press the left palm against the right palm without moving your hands. Feel the connection of the left arm through the left shoulder blade, the oblique muscles of the trunk (serratus anterior and internal obliques on the left, external obliques on the right) to the right side of the pelvis. Stop pressing and repeat the movement on the opposite diagonal. Repeat several times on each side, then press both palms together and feel the activation of both diagonals.

What to keep in mind: Good body alignment; hold the hands above the lower half of the sternum.

TIPS FOR PROS

If you would like to feel the activation more vividly, press more with the pinky side of the hand. You will feel the connection more vividly via the back arm lines to the shoulder blade and from there to the spiral line.

⚚ PILATES

ON ALL FOURS PRESSING THE CALVES INTO THE FLOOR TO ACTIVATE THE DEEP AND SUPERFICIAL ABDOMINAL MUSCLES AS WELL AS PRESSING WITH THE HANDS TO ACTIVATE THE OBLIQUE ABDOMINALS

Goal: Consciously activating the different parts of the abdominal muscles using the arms and legs.

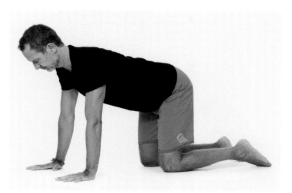

Starting position: Neutral all-fours position (see orientation and alignment).

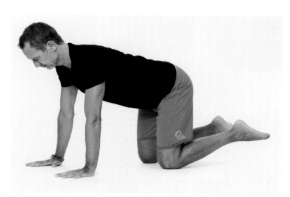

Execution: As you inhale, lift your calves and pointed feet off the floor.

As you exhale, begin by pressing the calves and tops of the feet back into the floor. Gradually increase pressure and feel the different layers of your abdominals being activated.

As you inhale, release the pressure and lift the calves and feet again.

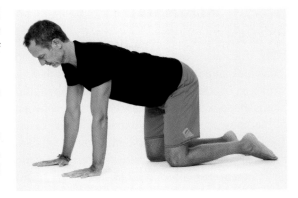

Then allow the calves to rest on the floor and begin pressing the palms into the floor, alternating hands. This is how you activate the oblique abdominal muscles.

Play with the movements to improve your activation awareness.

What to keep in mind: Good body alignment; elbows are extended but not locked.

TIPS FOR PROS

If you would like to feel the activation of abdominal muscles via the arms more vividly, press more with the pinkie-side of your hand. The more you press the calves into the mat, the more abdominal muscles are activated. Activation goes from the inside (transverse abdominals) to the outside (rectus abdominis).

3.1.3 ALIGNMENT

The term *alignment* refers to the orientation of multiple segments in a line. With respect to the human body, this means the ideal positioning of the joints relative to each other as well as the alignment of individual joint partners relative to each other. Successful alignment results in postural control with a minimum of strength effort and energy expenditure in stationary positions as well as during movement. This is made possible by balanced tension between the front and back of the body, the left and right half of the body, as well as the upper and lower extremities. This involves much more than muscle balance. The CNS (central nervous system) requires reliable information about the body's position and movement in space, the relationship between certain segments of the body to each other, and how gravity and environment can affect movement (Barth, 2005). Body awareness is thus an important criterion for optimal alignment. Only the interplay between proprioception and a balanced state of muscle tension or tonicity enables an economical movement sequence. The result is a feeling of lightness that people around you see as good posture and elegant movement.

ALIGNMENT IN THE STARTING POSITION

Correct body alignment is the foundation of every exercise. The exercise can only be successful if the body is placed in an optimal starting position. The term tensegrity, referring to pre-stressed tension (also see chapter 3.1.2 Centering) comes up with increasing frequency in this context. The word combination stems from the words tension = tensile stress and integrity = cohesion, an architectural model that involves the array of elastic and dimensionally stable elements. That is also how we can think of the body: the bones form dimensionally stable structures that maintain tension and are thereby kept at a distance via the elastic connective tissue. None of the bones touch and equal tension from all directions creates a flexible and simultaneously stable, reactive construct. But this also makes clear that minute changes to, or displacements of, one element always affect the entire structure. For instance, if one foot is not properly aligned while standing and is in a slightly pronated position, this misalignment can continue in the upper joints like knee, hip, pelvis, spine, and shoulder girdle and cause problems and pain.

Even though the above title says "starting position," it must be said that there are really no motionless positions. The body as a living organism is always in motion. Even if they are just micro-movements, they do permanently change the tension relationships; the body immediately reacts to the smallest weight shifts and continuously adapts to the new circumstance, sometimes triggered by just looking in another direction.

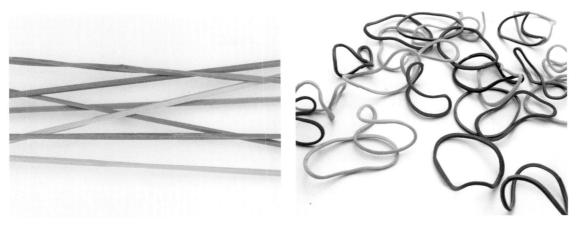

Figure 7: The bones as dimensionally stable elements maintain tension via the connective tissue. Equal tension from all directions creates both a stable and flexible system that is always reactive.

ALIGNMENT DURING AN EXERCISE

Alignment is of course maintained throughout the exercise sequence. This is probably the biggest challenge: optimal body tension in every position and during movement. The more complex the movement sequence, the more strength-intensive a position (e.g., push-ups or side planks), the more challenging it is to maintain lightness. It requires primarily good body awareness, functioning proprioception. Mechanoreceptor function in particular ensures that the participants are in alignment not just in space but also in their own bodies, and receive feedback about their posture and their body image via different tensions and forces. Exercises that emphasize body awareness, self-awareness, and embodiment are just as relevant to training as exercises that promote strength, mobility, or other exercise-related motor skills. Exercises that emphasize body awareness can also be used to teach basic anatomical knowledge and basic physiological relationships, and illustrate movement regularities. Understanding the array of dimensionally stable elements—meaning the construction of the skeleton, the position of the hip joints, construction of the shoulder girdle, the number of vertebrae, or the shape of the pelvis—their function, and interplay promotes an understanding of movement and thus a continuously improving movement technique.

Following are exercises that prepare all six basic positions (standing, seated, supine, prone, all-fours position, side-lying position).

STANDING ALIGNMENT

TAPPING

Goal: Activating and improving body awareness; knowledge about and overview of the body's construction, or rather achieving and refining positions.

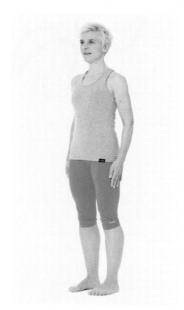

Starting position: Upright standing position; feet are hip-width apart; arms are relaxed.

Execution: Smooth out or tap the body with both hands. When smoothing the body, the hands are relaxed and the palms run over the skin or clothing. Tapping is done with slightly cupped hands and you can hear a faint, high tapping sound created by the air between the palm and the skin. Both forms of execution are more vigorous than tentative.

Smooth out the jaws.

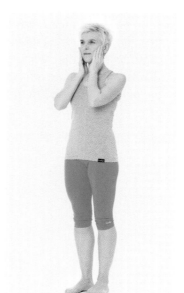

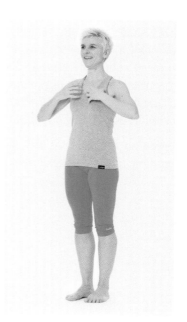

Smooth out the collarbones; tap the sternum.

Smooth out the front and rear costal arches.

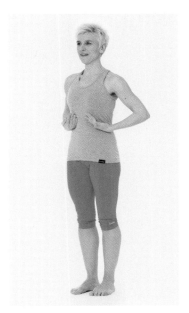
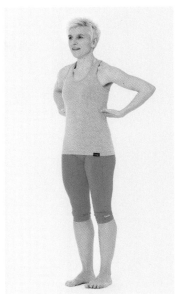

Smooth out the front and back of the iliac crest.

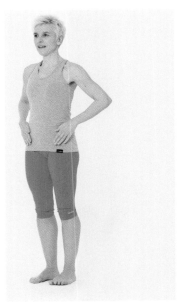
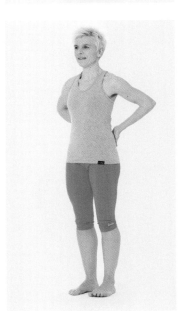

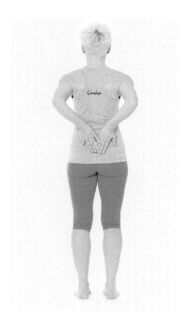

Tap the sacrum.

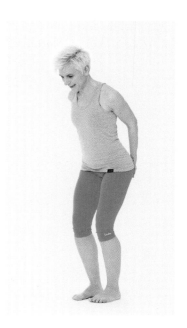

Smooth out the sit bones.

Tap the calves and thighs.

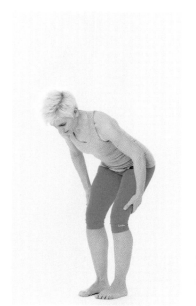

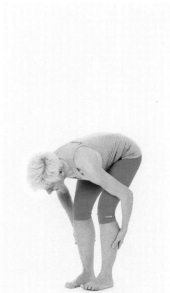

Smooth out the ankles, tops of the feet, toes, heels, Achilles tendons, calves, and back of the knees.

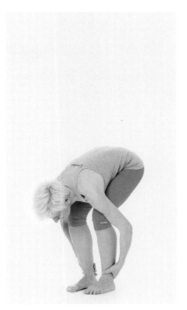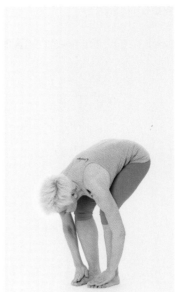

Tap and smooth out the hands and arms.

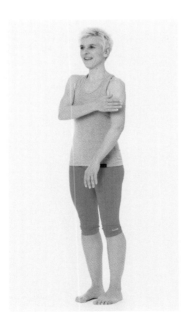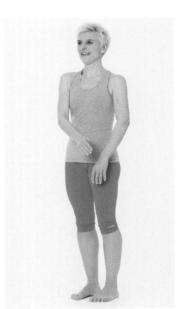

WEIGHT SHIFT

Goal: Feeling the feet's contact area with the floor and weigh shift.

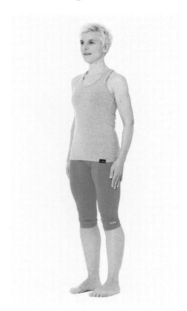

Starting position: Upright standing position; legs are parallel and feet are hip-width apart.

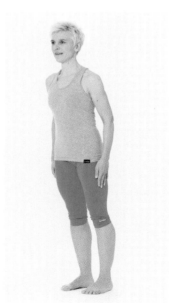
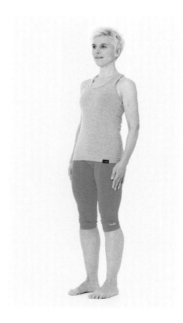

Execution: Shift your weight forward and back and slowly alternate rolling from the balls of the feet to the heels and back again. Notice how the tension at the front or back of the body changes, making sure the feet maintain contact with the floor and keep you from falling over. Imagine your body getting longer with each repetition and the head reaching up higher and higher.

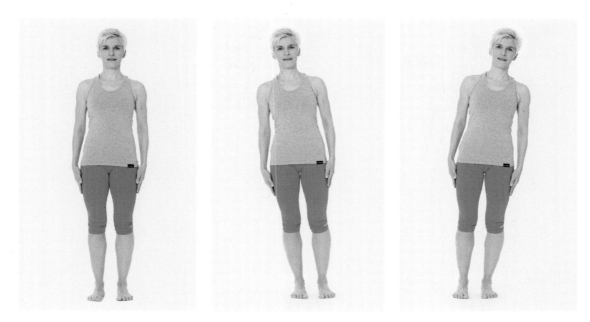

Now repeat the same pattern, moving side to side. The weight now shifts to the outside and inside edge of the foot; tension in the side body (lateral lines) changes and keeps you from falling to the side.

PLEASE NOTE

Feet hip-width apart means that an imaginary third foot would fit between your two feet.

TIP FOR INSTRUCTORS

To be able to keep an eye on large groups and correct them if necessary, it helps to have a broad view and scan the group. In doing so, the focus is on the silhouette of the matching joints or paired structures in the body (e.g., shoulders, iliac crest, gluteal folds, or kneecaps). This scan makes it easier to keep an overview and is done from three sides (front and back of the body, profile).

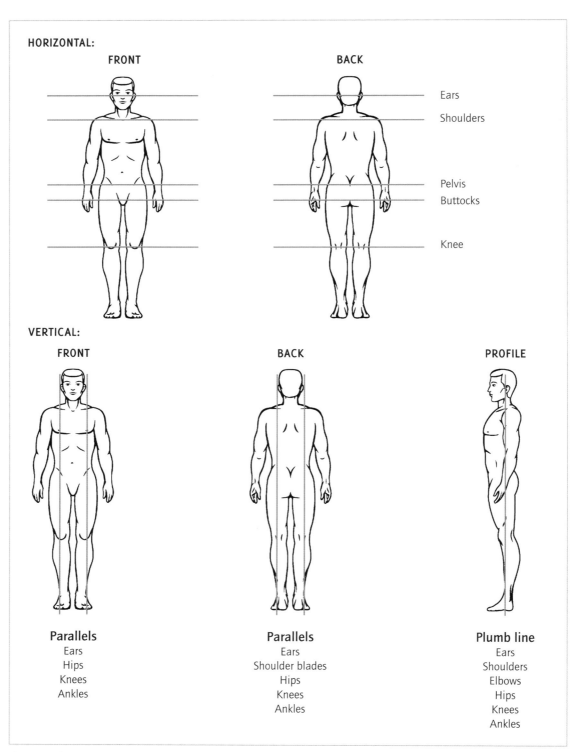

HORIZONTAL:

FRONT   BACK

Ears
Shoulders

Pelvis
Buttocks

Knee

VERTICAL:

FRONT   BACK   PROFILE

Parallels   **Parallels**   **Plumb line**
Ears   Ears   Ears
Hips   Shoulder blades   Shoulders
Knees   Hips   Elbows
Ankles   Knees   Hips
                         Ankles   Knees
                                                 Ankles

Figure 8: Quick body scan

SEATED ALIGNMENT

Goal: Finding the optimal position for the pelvis.

Starting position: Seated on the floor; feet are planted and hands rest on knees.

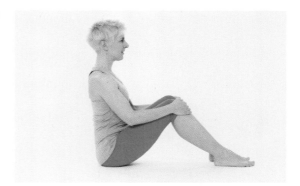

Execution: As you inhale, sit up tall by pushing the head up. As you exhale, tilt the pelvis back. The pubic bone pulls towards the navel, the low back is rounded and the sit bones point towards the heels. The gaze is forward and slightly down.

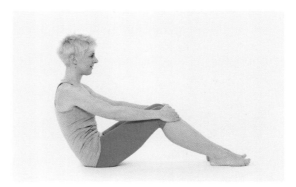

As you inhale, return the spine to an upright position and reposition the pelvis so the sit bones point to the floor. The sternum is lifted. Notice the position of the sit bones. They provide orientation for an upright seat. Repeat several times and notice how the sit bones point forward once and backward once. Then center the pelvis so the sit bones point down and the lumbar spine is in its natural lordotic curve.

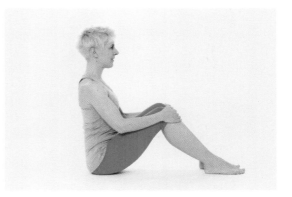

TIP FOR INSTRUCTORS

You can use your arms to help you move into the upright position by gripping the knees with your hands.

ALIGNMENT IN SUPINE POSITION 1

Goal: Finding the optimal position for the pelvis.

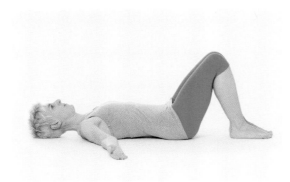

Starting position: On your back; feet are planted hip-width apart; arms rest on the floor in T-position; sit bones point towards the heels.

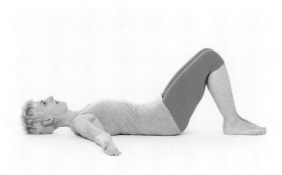

Execution: As you inhale, tilt the pelvis back. The pubic bone pulls towards the navel, the low back sinks into the floor, and the sit bones point towards the calves/ back of the knees.

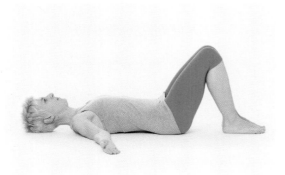

As you exhale, abruptly relax the pelvis so it drops back into its natural position with a slight post-pulse. Now the sit bones point towards the heels again.

PLEASE NOTE

The final position in which the pelvis drops into a relaxed position is the starting position for all subsequent exercises done in a supine position.

ALIGNMENT IN SUPINE POSITION 2

Goal: Creating alignment in the shoulder girdle.

Starting position: On your back; feet are planted hip-width apart; arms are extended towards the ceiling with palms facing each other.

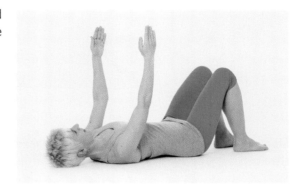

Execution: As you inhale, extend your hands to the ceiling, opening the shoulder blades. The nape of the neck remains long and the shoulders low.

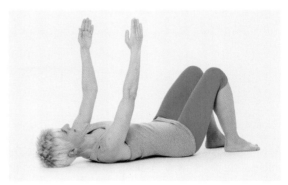

As you exhale, allow the shoulder blades to abruptly drop to the floor.

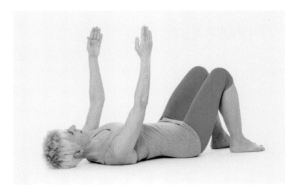

ALIGNMENT IN PRONE POSITION

Goal: Build alignment in pelvis and ribcage.

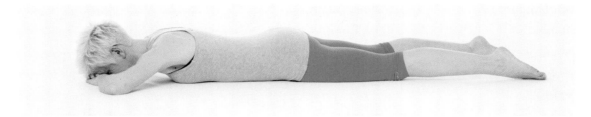

Starting position: On your stomach; the forehead rests on the hands; the shoulder girdle is wide, the shoulders are low.

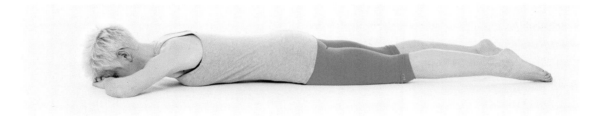

Execution: As you inhale, allow the breath to flow underneath the costal arches, causing them to widen.

As you exhale, the lower costal arches slide into the body; the abdominal wall rests against the low back and gently pulls away from the floor. The pubic bone sinks into the floor.

PLEASE NOTE

The shoulder girdle stays wide and relaxed. The elbows pull slightly to the outside.

ALL-FOURS POSITION 1

Goal: Build alignment in the shoulder girdle.

Starting position: On all fours, palms are below shoulders; knees are below hips; the crown of the head points forward; the tailbone points to the back; the elbows face each other, and the middle fingers point forward.

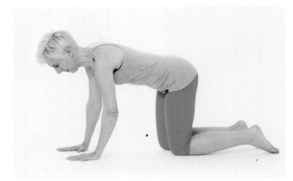

Execution: As you inhale, the shoulder blades move towards each other. The sternum moves towards the floor, the elbows remain long, and the pelvis is stable.

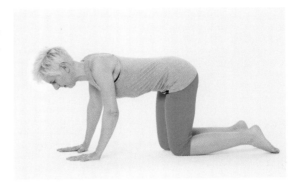

As you exhale, press your hands into the floor so the shoulder blades move apart again.

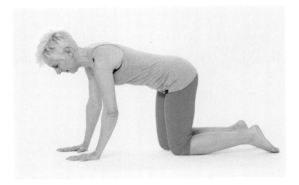

IMPORTANT

Cervical spine alignment with respect to its length remains the same during the entire exercise sequence. All of the movement takes place in the upper back.

ALL-FOURS POSITION 2

Goal: Build alignment in the pelvic girdle

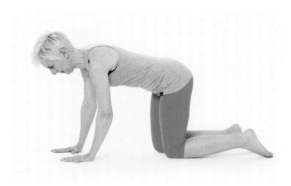

Starting position: On all fours, palms are below shoulders; knees are below hips; the crown of the head points forward; the tailbone points to the back; the elbows face each other, and the middle fingers point forward.

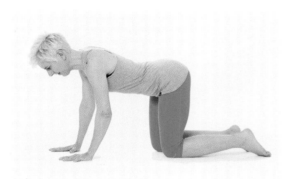

Execution: As you inhale, tilt the pelvis forward so the back is slightly arched. The sit bones now point diagonally back and up.

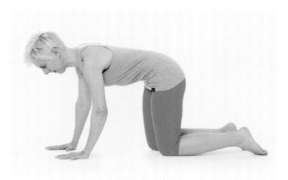

As you exhale, tilt the pelvis back and round the lumbar spine.

Repeat this several times and notice that the sit bones alternately point diagonally back and towards the back of the knees. Next, center the pelvis so the sit bones point back and the lumbar spine is in its natural lordotic curve.

IMPORTANT

Alignment of the shoulder girdle in terms of its length is maintained throughout the exercise sequence. All of the movement takes place in the pelvis and lower back.

ALIGNMENT IN A SIDE-LYING POSITION

Goal: Build alignment in the pelvic girdle and spine.

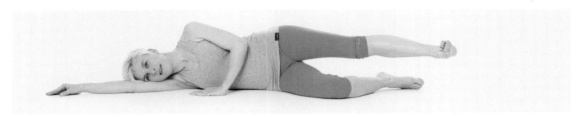

Starting position: While on your side, the bottom arm is extended, and the top arm rests in front of the body. The upper hand is propped on the floor at chest level; the bottom knee is bent; the top leg is extended and lifted to hip level; the foot is flexed (dorsal flexion; pull the top of the foot towards the body); back of the head, thoracic spine, sacrum, and feet are lined up; shoulders and pelvis are lined up vertically.

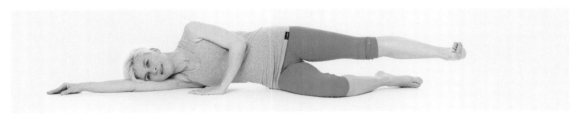

Execution: As you exhale, push out through the heel; the pelvis rolls on the greater trochanter and the lower waist and lower ribs lift off the floor. A small gap appears below the waist. The iliac crests are stacked.

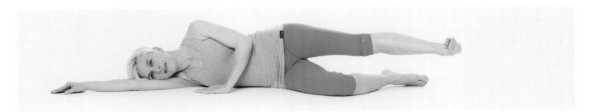

As you inhale, the pelvis rolls back into the starting position and the lower waist lowers back down to the floor. Repeat several times.

PLEASE NOTE

The final position, in which the waist has lifted away from the floor, is the starting position for all subsequent side-lying exercises.

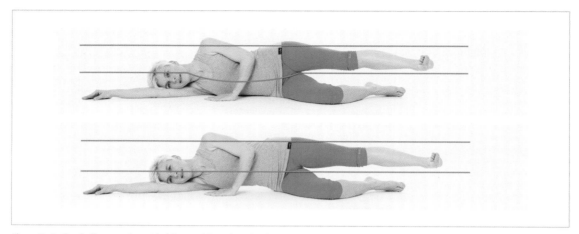

Figure 9: Optimal alignment in a side-lying position. The spine is parallel to the floor; both sides of the body are nearly symmetrical.

IMPORTANT

The spine remains straight, meaning not flexing, extending, or leaning forward or back. It merely lengthens from a slight lateral flexion in the starting position, meaning parallel to the floor.

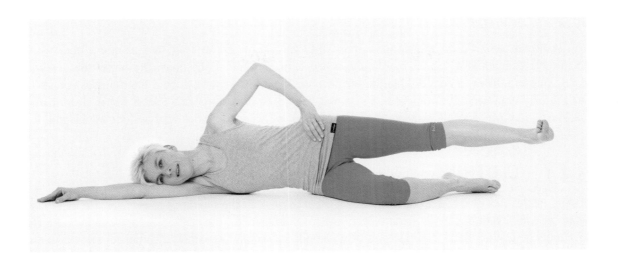

TIP FOR STUDENTS

The student places the upper hand against the upper iliac crest for support and directs the pelvis.

TIP FOR INSTRUCTORS

The instructors can recognize the correct execution if both sides of the waist are equally long in the final position, meaning the distance between the upper iliac crest and the bottom costal arch is the same.

3.2   GEAR

You would like to start doing Pilates and wonder what you might need. We want to make your introduction to the Pilates method a success by offering a few basic tips and suggestions. The better the general conditions and the more comfortable you will feel, the more you will enjoy doing the exercises and stick with it long-term. Regardless of where the training is held, be it at home, at a Pilates studio, at a fitness facility, or at a gym, a small assortment of clothing and equipment, and the right attitude are helpful.

3.2.1   CLOTHING

Joseph Pilates most likely did not worry about what to wear in the mornings to exercise. He generally wore the same types of clothes. Regardless of the temperature, he wore black, gray, or white gym shorts. His upper body was usually bare. Occasionally, he added a very tight t-shirt or a turtleneck sweater, both white. He, of course, exercised barefoot or, depending on the surface, he might have worn gymnastics slippers. The women at his studio wore tight gymnastics clothing, and some were quite scantily clad by today's standards in bikini-like suits.

Choose comfortable attire that allows you to move freely. Form-fitting clothes that show the contours of the body allow you and your instructors to better evaluate your execution of movements. Thick seams or zippers that may cause pressure points are not a good choice.

Pilates is a barefoot form of exercise. It is a way to also exercise the feet and ensures our feet's functional sensitivity. However, you can certainly wear socks or gymnastics slippers for hygiene or medical reasons. Socks with non-slip soles are a good choice to prevent slipping.

A towel to place on top of the mat and a second one to dry off perspiration or to use for cushioning during some exercises round out the necessary gear.

3.2.2   EQUIPMENT

Practice on a comfortable thick mat. Use towels or small pillows for cushioning. Aids like the Pilates ball, the Pilates foam roller, or an elastic band (see program section) help users to better understand the movements and to master them. For exercise programs that use small props you will need an elastic band, a roller, and a Pilates ball.

3.2.3 ENVIRONMENT

To practice, choose a space that is well ventilated, light, quiet, and not too cold. It should have enough room for you to execute the movements. Avoid direct light from above. It will blind you during exercises in a supine position.

3.2.4 MENTAL ATTITUDE

Build a specific timeslot for your Pilates workout into your day. Shut out any outside interferences as best you can. Practice with focus and dedication. Pilates is not something that works "on the side." Turn off the television, radio, and stereo. Be patient and hold a positive dialog with yourself. No one is born a master.

Begin with a short program. Carefully look at the exercise sequence and memorize it. This will allow you to fully focus on the execution during your practice.

Take time for the basics. If you are sloppy here, you won't master the more advanced exercises.

3.2.5 INSTRUCTOR

Find a competent instructor. The German Pilates Association, as well as their associated training institutions, have lists of graduates and are happy to suggest an instructor near you. Regular external monitoring to prevent inaccuracies from creeping into your execution is always an advantage. One sign of a good instructor is that he will keep an eye on the group during the entire practice, and frequently changes places to be able to issue detailed corrections to individuals and the group as a whole. An instructor who only participates in the workout and announces the exercises will not help you make progress. A good instructor can also help when you have questions or problems with the exercises. Often a minor modification or specific tip is enough to make the exercise work. That is also why you will find lots of tips and suggestions in this book, which are always color-coded. An experienced instructor is part of a network and in cases of physical problems is able to suggest the appropriate contact person or knows where to find the necessary information.

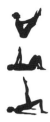

4 EXERCISES

4.1 PREPARATORY EXERCISES

Before getting started with the traditional exercises and exercise programs, we will introduce some of the most important pre-Pilates exercises. As the name suggests, they will be practiced beforehand and serve as the foundation for the original Pilates exercises or for independent practice at home. At an even more advanced level, the pre-Pilates exercises are well suited as building exercises or to start off a class.

4.1.1 BASIC BRIDGING

Goal: Spinal articulation, control of hamstring muscles, alignment particularly of the lower extremities or mechanical axes, abdominal strength.

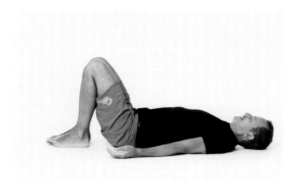

Starting position: On your back; feet are planted, heels are below knee joints; legs are hip-width apart; arms rest alongside the body.

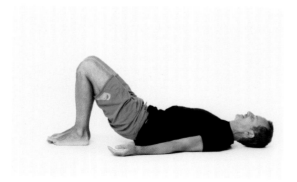

Execution: As you exhale, roll the spine up vertebrae by vertebrae, starting at the tailbone; sit bones pull towards the back of the knees. Your weight rests on your shoulder girdle.

Inhale, and as you exhale again, incrementally roll back down into the neutral pelvic position starting at the sternum.

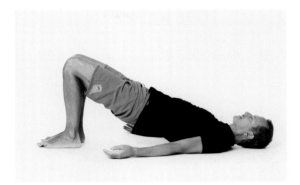

Variations: Take several breaths to roll back down; stay in shoulder bridge and rotate the pelvis or push it to the side; roll up or down next to the spine.

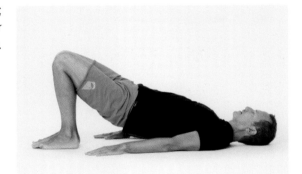

What to pay attention to: The legs remain parallel (a frequent mistake is the splaying out of the knees); keep the cervical spine long as you roll down; weight rests on the shoulder girdle (between the shoulder blades) and not on the cervical spine; maintain integration of ribs and pelvis.

TIPS FOR PROS

This exercise should be a part of every Pilates class, even an advanced class. Continue to find new variations to keep it exciting and appealing (e.g., shifting the trunk to the side or rotating it around its vertical axis, rolling up and down on one leg).

The basic bridge frequently causes hamstring cramps. If this happens, briefly interrupt the exercise and loosen up the legs. When resuming the exercise, make sure to activate the abdominal and pelvic floor muscles prior to the first pelvic tilt.

4.1.2   LOW ABS

Goal: Activating the abdominal muscles, stabilizing the neutral pelvic position.

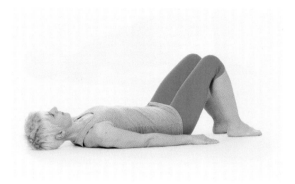

Starting position: On your back, feet are planted, legs are hip-width apart; arms rest alongside the body.

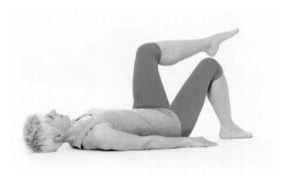

Execution: As you exhale, gently pull the abdominal wall inward and lift one knee towards the upper body.

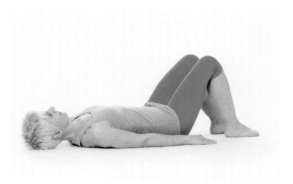

Now inhale again, and with the next exhale lower the leg back down to starting position. Repeat, alternating sides.

Variation 1: As you exhale, lift one knee at a time towards the upper body until the backs of both thighs are parallel to the floor. As you exhale, lower the legs back down one at a time.

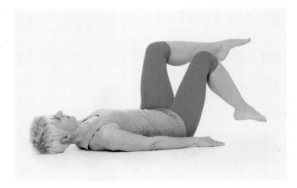

Variation 2: As you exhale, lift both knees towards the body until the backs of the thighs are parallel to the floor. With your next exhale, simultaneously lower both legs back down to the floor.

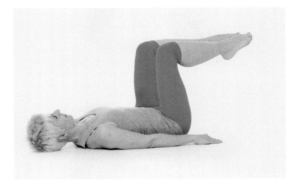

What to pay attention to: Lifting and lowering the legs is a fluid motion; shoulders and nape stay relaxed. The abdominal wall should remain flat during the entire movement sequence and the pelvis remains still. If the rectus abdominis muscles suddenly pop up or the pelvis tilts forward (arched back), you should hold off on these variations and work on centering.

TIPS FOR PROS

This exercise will show you if your participants have understood the centering principle and are able to apply it.

4.1.3 HALF ROLL BACK

Goal: Articulating and mobilizing the lumbar spine, strengthening the abdominal and pelvic floor muscles.

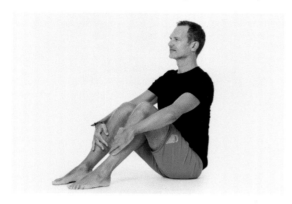

Starting position: Neutral seated position; feet are planted hip-width apart; hands lightly hold on to the shins.

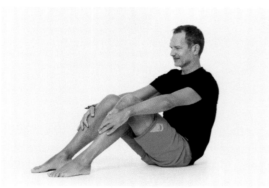

Execution: As you inhale, lift the spine and reach for the ceiling with the crown of the head. As you exhale, pull the abdominal wall inward and tilt the pelvis back until the spine forms a letter C. The gaze is forward and down and the arms are extended.

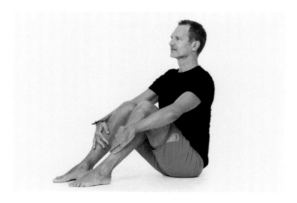

As you inhale, straighten up again, leading with the head, to return to the starting position.

Variation: Arms are extended next to the thighs, palms face inward. Roll down until the sacrum rests on the floor. With the next exhalation, roll up again by reaching forward with your fingers.

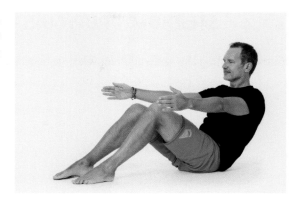

What to pay attention to: The spine is long during the entire exercise sequence, the C-shape is even, and the shoulder girdle stays wide open.

TIPS FOR PROS

Hold the rolling-down motion and add little pulses towards the sacrum and lumbar spine; add a spinal rotation.

4.1.4 STERNUM DROP/CURL-UP

Goal: Activating the abdominal muscles, stabilizing the neutral pelvic position.

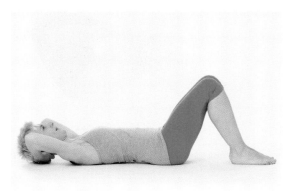

Starting position: On your back, feet are planted, legs are hip-width apart, hands are folded at the back of the head; elbows are slightly raised so the shoulder girdle can remain open.

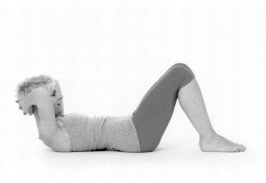

Execution: As you exhale, gently pull the abdominal wall inward; the lower costal arches sink into the body. Roll up head and shoulders.

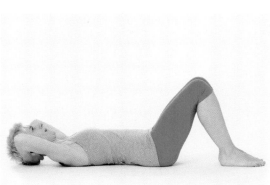

With your next exhalation, actively release and roll back down into starting position.

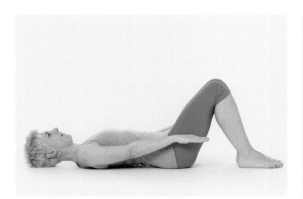 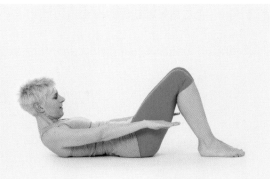

Variation: The arms are extended alongside the body at thigh level and reach towards the feet.

What to pay attention to: The pelvis remains in a neutral position; the head is cradled in the palms (avoid pulling up with the hands).

TIPS FOR PROS

Before rolling up, gently lengthen the cervical spine and let the sternum relax and drop between the shoulder blades.

This exercise is the prerequisite for all exercises during which the head and shoulders are rolled up (e.g., one hundred, double-leg stretch, single-leg stretch) and prevents muscle tension in the neck, shoulders, and nape area.

4.1.5   SCAPULAR REACH

Goal: Mobilizing the shoulder joints and shoulder blades, relaxing the shoulder and neck muscles.

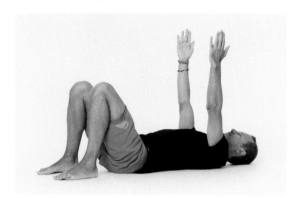

Starting position: On your back, feet are planted, legs are hip-width apart, arms are extended to the ceiling, palms face inward.

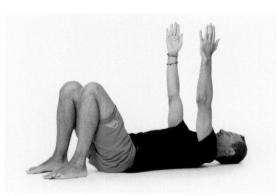

Execution: As you inhale, reach for the ceiling with the arms. Shoulder blades spread apart and lift off the floor. The head remains on the floor, the cervical spine stays long.

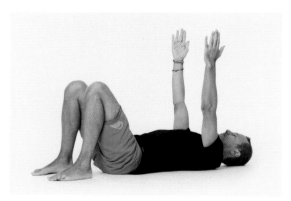

As you exhale, let the shoulder blades come back down to the floor.

Variation: Reach for the ceiling with only one arm at a time while turning the head in the opposite direction.

Instead of allowing the arms to slide back into the starting position, let them drop.

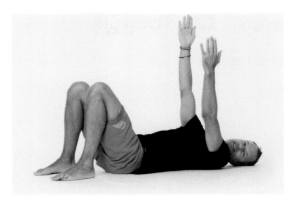

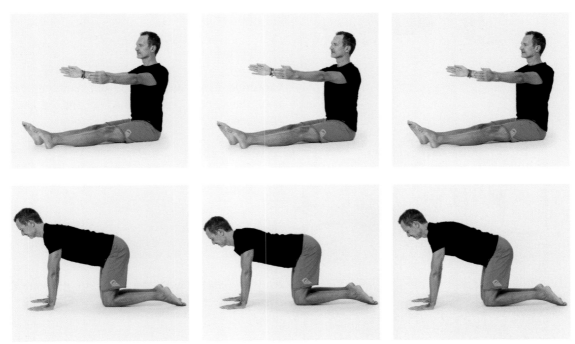

Additional variations: Spreading the shoulder blades or pulling them forward (protraction) and squeezing them together (retraction) can also be practiced in other starting positions (standing, seated, on all fours). This allows participants to generalize the movement pattern.

What to pay attention to: Relax the jaw. Pelvis and legs do not move.

TIPS FOR PROS

Performing this exercise on the Pilates foam roller allows the shoulder blades to come even closer to the floor.

4.1.6 CAT STRETCH

Goal: Mobilizing the spine, controlling alignment in the shoulder and pelvic girdle in a supporting position.

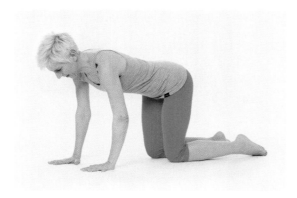

Starting position: On all fours, shoulders are stacked over wrists and hips are stacked over knees. The spine is in natural alignment.

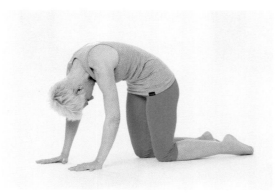

Execution: As you exhale, press your hands into the floor. The tailbone points to the floor and the spine is rounded.

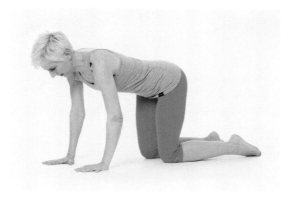

As you inhale, return the spine to its neutral position.

Variation: Instead of rounding (flexing) the spine, move it into extension (arch the back), whereby hands and knees pull towards each other and the crown of the head and tailbone pull as far away from each other as possible.

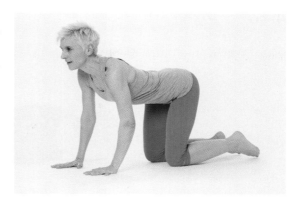

What to pay attention to: For an optimal supporting or starting position, the elbows face inward, palms press into the floor, and the shoulder girdle is wide open. Spinal flexion is even and shoulder-girdle alignment is maintained during flexion.

TIPS FOR PROS

To evenly flex the spine, gently pull the abdominal wall in and up (pushing it against the wall of the low back). The lower costal arches slide into the body to facilitate the transition from lumbar to thoracic spine.

PLEASE NOTE

Participants often complain of wrist pain during supporting poses. This is primarily a result of a lack of shoulder-girdle arrangement and insufficient shoulder-girdle alignment. In this case, it is best to shorten the length of the pose and do fewer repetitions, and insert other exercises that don't require wrist support.

4.1.7   DART

Goal: Extension of the thoracic spine, centering in a supine position.

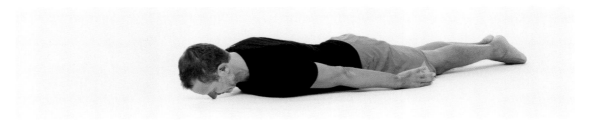

Starting position: On your stomach, the arms are extended alongside the body, thumbs pointing down; the tailbone is slightly tucked; the pubic bone sinks into the floor.

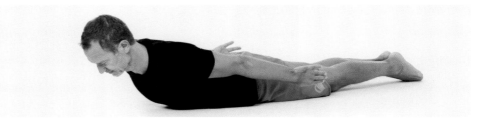

Execution: As you exhale, reach with your hands towards your feet. The thoracic spine lengthens and the upper body lifts slightly off the floor. The gaze is down and very slightly forward, depending on the extension of the thoracic spine.

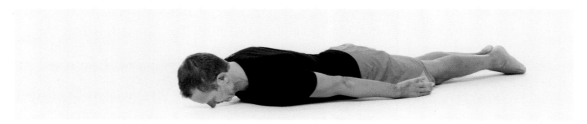

As you inhale, lower the upper body back down to the floor while maintaining spinal extension.

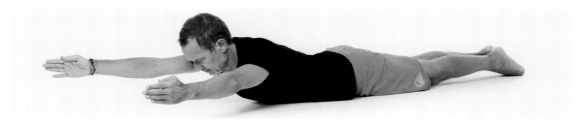

Variation: Arms are extended forward or up during extension of the thoracic spine.

What to pay attention to: Maintain extension of the cervical and lumbar spine (no excessive lordotic curvature); hips are extended.

TIPS FOR PROS

Maintain spinal extension while performing different arm movements (e.g., floating arms, unilateral or bilateral). Perform the exercise with arms extended forward (progression with a longer lever).

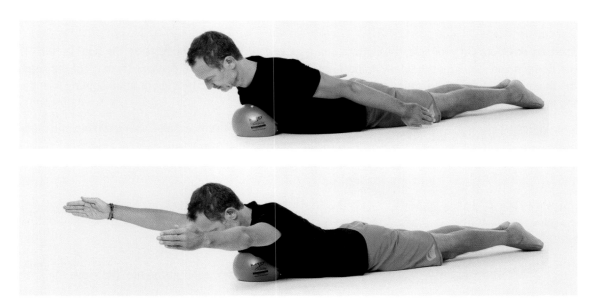

Participants with severe rounding of the thoracic spine (kyphosis) or tight chest muscles have trouble lying on their stomachs. Suggest placing a wobble cushion or something similar under the chest. Large-breasted women can also find a supine position uncomfortable. Suggest an all-fours pose (see Cat stretch) or a supine position on a step to avoid pressure on the chest.

4.1.8 SIDE KICK PREPARATION

Goal: Trunk stability and overall alignment, segmented hip movement, controlling the mechanical axis.

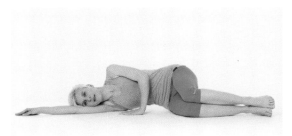 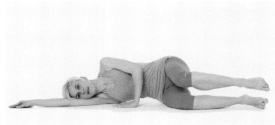

Starting position: On your side, the bottom arm is extended. The top hand rests on the floor in front of the sternum and stabilizes the side-lying posture; legs and hips are bent 90 degrees; the back of the head, the thoracic spine, and the sacrum are lined up along the back edge of the mat or an imaginary line; the top leg is raised to hip level.

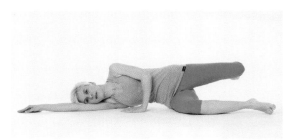

Execution: As you exhale, extend the hip and move the top leg back.

As you inhale, bend at the hip and move the knee forward again.

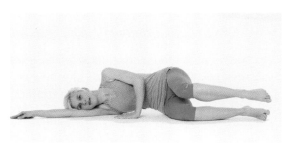

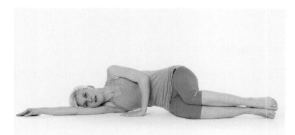 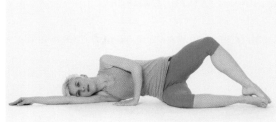

Variation 1: Legs are stacked and the top thigh opens (external hip rotation) and closes while the feet touch.

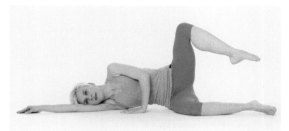 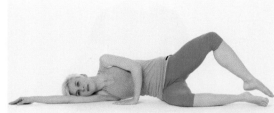

Variation 2: The upper thigh circles from the hip joint.

What to pay attention to: The pelvis remains steady. Maintain the distance on both sides between the iliac crest and lower costal arches (maintain distance between bottom side of waist and floor); shoulder girdle is steady with shoulders stacked.

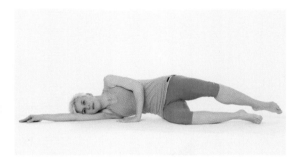

TIPS FOR PROS

For a bigger challenge, extend the top arm to the ceiling during the exercise sequence.

Side-lying exercises are challenging because support from the floor surface is reduced and is asymmetrical, and the movement takes place behind the body, and thus outside of the field of vision. The instructor can stand behind the participant and stabilize the lumbar spine with one leg for support. The participant should imagine lying with his back against a wall.

4.1.9   SIDE BEND

Goal: Mobilizing the spine along the sagittal plane, arranging the shoulder girdle.

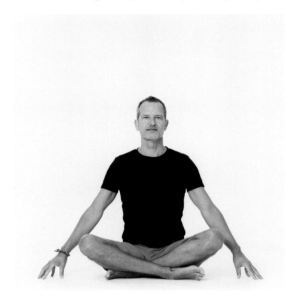

Starting position: Sit on the floor with legs crossed and arms extended at the sides.

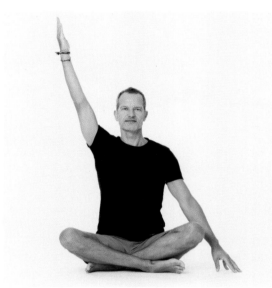
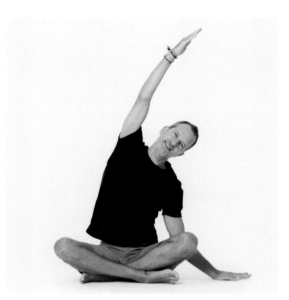

Execution: As you inhale, lift the spine. As you exhale, laterally raise the right arm and then sweep it up and extend it overhead and to the opposite side in an arc. The spine bends to the left, the left elbow is bent, and the left hand rests on the floor for support.

As you inhale, return to the starting position.

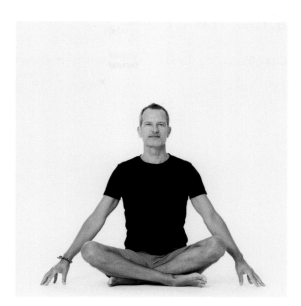

Variation: Dynamic side bends from one side to the other. Use the supporting hand to push off and the other hand for a soft landing.

What to pay attention to: The neck stays long, and the shoulder blades maintain contact with the back costal arches; both sit bones maintain contact with the floor; all movement takes place on the sagittal plane.

TIPS FOR PROS

Press the supporting hand into the floor and open the upper costal arches to the ceiling to intensify the side bend (lateral flexion).

During this exercise, the pelvis likes to tilt forward (anterior tilt; arched back) and the ribs push forward. Therefore, make sure the ribcage stays over the pelvis and doesn't push forward.

4.1.10 TWIST

Goal: Mobilizing the spine in the transverse plane; arranging the shoulder girdle.

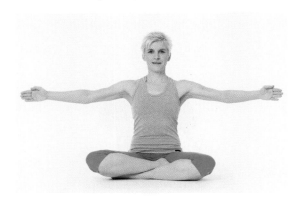

Starting position: Sit on the floor with legs crossed and arms extended to the sides at shoulder level. Palms face forward.

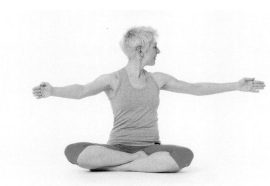

Execution: As you inhale, sit up tall. As you exhale, rotate the spine around its vertical axis and look in the direction of rotation.

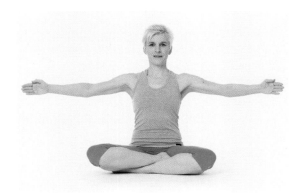

As you inhale, return to the starting position.

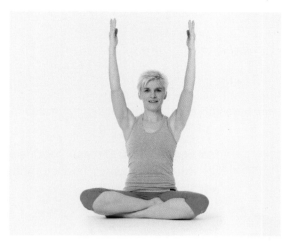 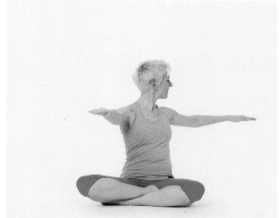

Variation 1: Extend the arms to the ceiling, then lower the arms horizontally to shoulder level as though you were trying to push the air down.

Variation 2: In the beginning, it is a good idea to shorten the arm lever to make sure the movement takes place strictly in the spine. To do so, cross the arms in front of the chest with the palms at a level with the pectoral muscles.

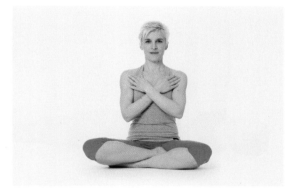

What to pay attention to: All the movement takes place on the transverse plane. Avoid shifting or bending the ribcage. Maintain alignment of the shoulder girdle, meaning only the spine moves, not the shoulders.

TIPS FOR PROS

Add small pulses at the end of a rotation. Do the exercise using light weights.

⚡ PILATES

4.2 TRADITIONAL EXERCISES

4.2.1 ONE HUNDRED

Goal: Activating the core, increasing stability and abdominal strength, coordination, increasing circulation, preparation and warm-up.

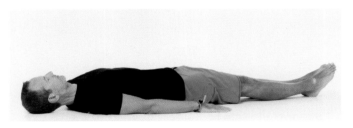

Starting position: On your back, legs are extended in closed position. Arms rest alongside the body.

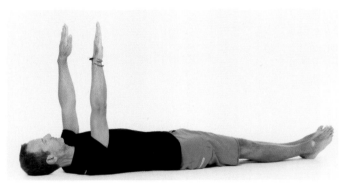

Execution: Extend the arms to the ceiling and get centered.

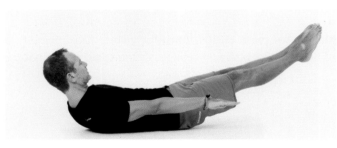

Then lower the arms to just above thigh-level, tuck the chin and roll up the upper body to the tips of the shoulder blades (lift the upper body and head until you can feel your upper abdominals engage).

As you lift the head and move the arms, also lift the legs; hold up head and legs equal distance from the floor, or lift the legs to a point you can manage.

Take 5 slow breaths through the nose and exhale 5x through the mouth or nose as you vigorously pump the arms up and down. Pump up to 100x, then lower the head, arms, and legs back down to the floor.

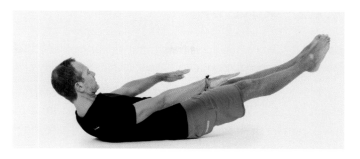

Variations: Legs remain extended on the floor; cushion the shoulder blades and head until you have sufficient strength to hold the head up; knees are bent and feet are planted; legs are raised 90/90 degrees; legs are extended to the ceiling at 45 degrees or more; begin with 20-30 repetitions; pump the arms higher above the floor; extend the arms towards the head and pump.

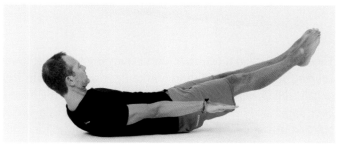

What to pay attention to: Stay centered throughout the entire movement sequence. The back maintains the same distance to the floor throughout the exercise; arms pump vigorously; hold the legs at one level.

TIPS FOR PROS

Choose an arm and leg position that is in line with your client's ability level. The breath flows slowly and evenly; abdominal muscles must be strong enough to support the legs and head throughout the entire movement sequence.

The client must be able to activate the upper abdomen to stabilize the head. This also supports the effort of the lower abdominal muscles as well as the back muscles. If this is not possible, the client will need support from a ball, a roller, a Pilates Arc, a spine corrector, or the instructor, until he has built up sufficient strength.

4.2.2   ROLL UP

Goal: Articulating the spine, improving spinal mobility, stretching the low back and back of the legs, teaches the concept of axial extension, increases stability and abdominal strength, coordination.

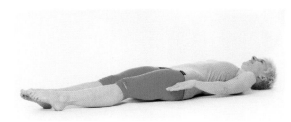

Starting position: On your back, legs are extended in a closed position or hip-width apart, arms extended alongside the body.

Execution: Extend the arms to the ceiling; as you exhale, lower the arms overhead as far as you can while keeping your back from lifting off the floor; as you inhale, extend the arms up over the shoulders; as you exhale, roll up vertebrae by vertebrae starting with the head until your sit bones press into the floor and your upper body is parallel to your legs; as you inhale, begin rolling back down in a controlled motion starting at the pelvis; as you exhale, continue to roll all the way down and extend the arms overhead again.

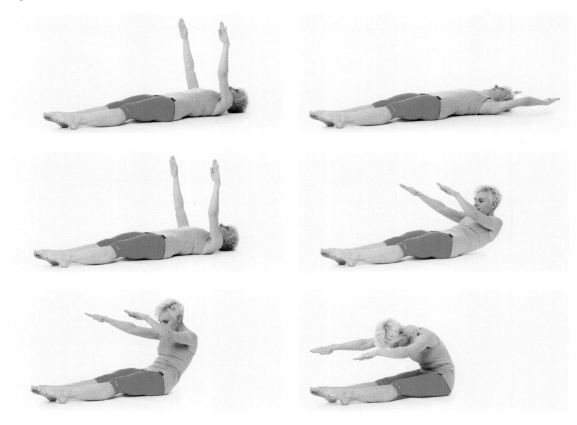

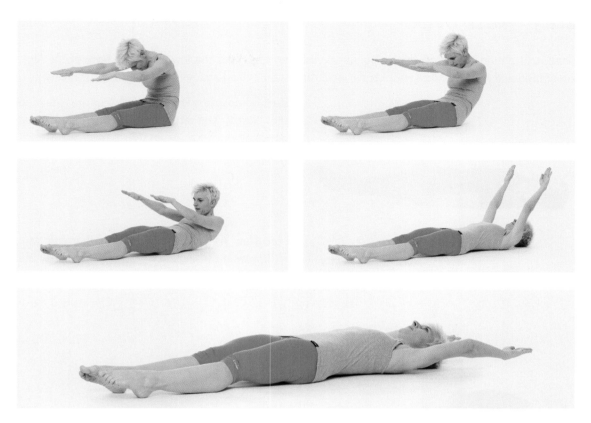

Variations: Both knees are bent and feet are planted; legs are raised in a 90/90-degree position and hands rest against the back of the thighs (assisted roll up).

What to pay attention to: For an even arch in the cervical spine, tuck the chin to the chest and not the throat. Create an even arch throughout the entire spine. The motion comes from the abdominal muscles; keep the feet or legs on the floor. Your abdominal muscles support your upper body during the forward bend. Don't allow the upper body to drop onto your legs. Stay centered throughout the entire movement sequence. The distance between your back and the floor does not change when the arms move towards the head (no arched back!).

TIPS FOR PROS

Look in the direction of movement, and lengthen the body. Use your stomach and not your arms to roll up. Work with your breath without using momentum. Cushion the spine in places where you are unable to make contact with the mat during the rolling motion. As you roll up, stick out your tongue or press it against your lower lip.

4.2.3 ROLL OVER

Goal: Articulating the spine, improving spinal mobility, stretching the low back and back of the legs, integrating and activating the entire body, increasing stability and abdominal strength, hip mobility.

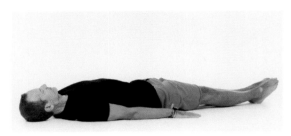

Starting position: On your back, legs are extended and closed; feet are gently pointed; arms rest alongside the body, palms down; fingertips stretch towards the feet.

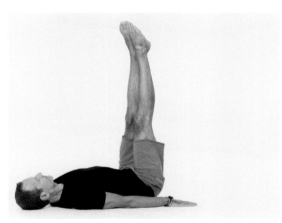

Execution: As you inhale, activate your core and lift the extended legs from the hips until they are perpendicular to the trunk.

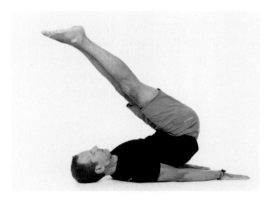 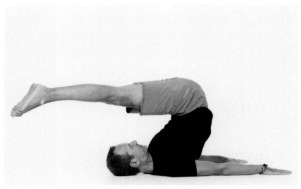

As you exhale, roll over vertebrae by vertebrae up to the shoulder blades. Actively push the toes towards the wall behind you and keep the abdominal wall low and flat as a counteraction. Your weight now rests on your shoulders.

As you inhale, open the legs to shoulder width.

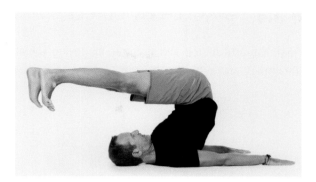

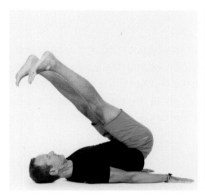 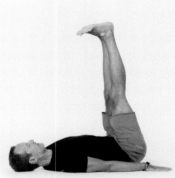 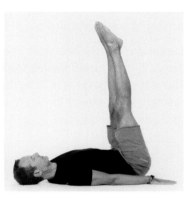

As you exhale, roll back down to the floor in a controlled motion, vertebrae by vertebrae. As you do so, allow the sternum to soften and keep your waist long and lifted. When your legs are once more perpendicular to the ceiling, finish by inhaling again. As you exhale, start the movement again. Repeat 3x, then roll up with legs shoulder-width apart and down with legs closed. Repeat 3x.

What to pay attention to: Only roll up to the shoulder blades, never onto the neck; tighten your abdominal muscles and keep the pelvis lifted. Control the weight of your legs and only roll back as far as you can stay in control; keep the sternum soft and the waist long to take pressure off the nape. Also use your arms to control the movement, but keep the shoulder blades on the floor. Create an even arch along the entire spine. The movement originates with the abdominal muscles. Stay centered and maintain axial extension throughout the entire movement sequence.

TIPS FOR PROS

Keep your eyes up on the ceiling and lengthen the body. Use your abs to roll up and your arms for support. Work with your breath without using momentum (particularly in the legs). Cushion your pelvis with a Pilates roller or something similar to create an easier starting position.

4.2.4 SINGLE-LEG CIRCLE

Goal: Hip articulation and strength, improving spinal stability, learning about the relationship between the lower extremities and the core; creating awareness of isolated joint movements, leg stretches.

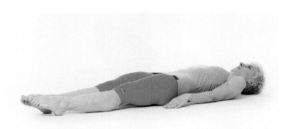

Starting position: On your back, legs are extended and open hip-width apart; feet are gently pointed; arms rest alongside the body with the palms down; fingertips reach towards the toes.

Execution: Pull the bent right knee into the chest and hold the shin (or the back of the thigh) with both hands. Gently stretch the leg towards the upper body for 2-3 breaths. Then extend the leg to the ceiling and place the hands as high on the leg as you can to deepen the stretch for another three breaths. Release the hands and extend the leg further towards the ceiling. As you inhale, guide the extended leg towards your nose. As you exhale, guide the leg towards the opposite shoulder and make a small circle with your

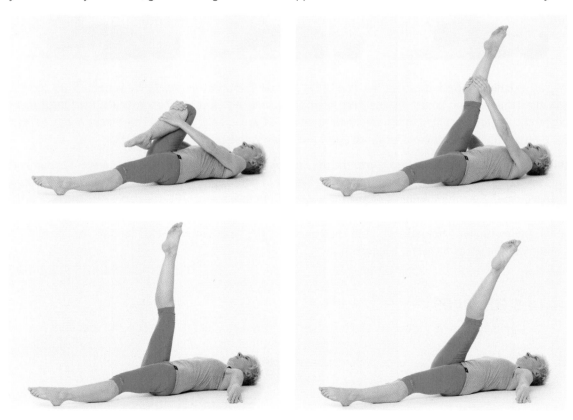

toes back to the starting position. Keep the pelvis steady and the body aligned on the floor. Complete five leg circles in this manner and then switch direction for another five circles. After you have finished circling in both directions, pull the knee into the chest again with both hands for a closing stretch.

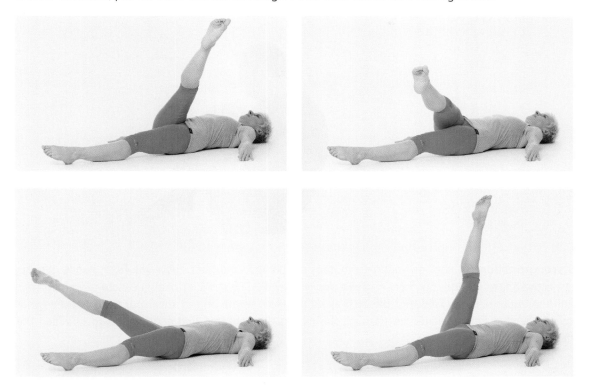

Variations: Bend the working leg and the supporting leg; make the circles bigger; lift the pelvis and rotate the upper body as the leg crosses the body.

What to pay attention to: Begin with small circles for more control; maintain body alignment throughout the entire movement; pull the toes up towards the ceiling while simultaneously allowing the femoral head to sink deep into the hip socket. Stay centered and maintain axial extension throughout the entire movement sequence.

TIPS FOR PROS

Your anchor points are the heel resting on the floor, the pelvis, ribcage, shoulder blades, arms, and the back of the head. Keep your eyes on the ceiling above you, create length in the body, use your abdominal muscles and only use your arms for support. Work controlled in time with your breath. Support your head with a pillow if needed. Begin by moving the supporting foot farther to the outside to increase the support surface and create more stability.

4.2.5 ROLLING LIKE A BALL/ROLLING BACK

Goal: Massaging the spine, improving balance, working on coordination via dynamic body movements, stretching the spine and opening the low back, improving coordinated use of abdominal strength.

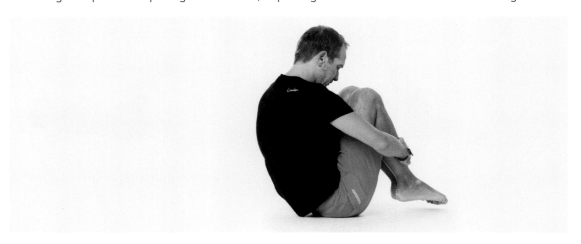

Starting position: Sit back on your sacrum; toes are pointed and float above the floor; hands grip the respective ankles (or right hand on left ankle and left hand on right ankle); heels are close to your bottom. Roll the upper body forward in a big arch as though you were trying to stick your head between your knees; the chin pulls towards the sternum; the elbows are bent and pull gently outward to widen the shoulders.

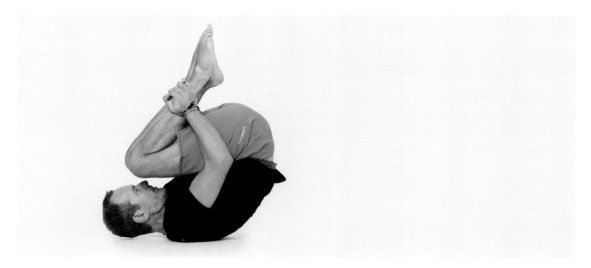

Execution: As you inhale, roll back to your shoulder blades. Keep your body in the ball shape. As you exhale, roll back to the starting position. Find your rolling and breathing rhythm.

Variations: Grip the back of your thighs. Hold this balance pose. Gather momentum with your legs to get a feel for the rolling motion. You can do a curl down if rolling isn't possible.

What to pay attention to: Keep your heels close to your bottom (no momentum); tuck the chin to the chest; hold the leg position; maintain a long arch in the spine (don't slouch in the low back) and keep the shoulders wide; when you roll back, actively pull the abdominal wall towards your back to take the weight off the nape; consciously roll on every vertebrae; head and feet remain off the ground.

TIPS FOR PROS

To find the sacral position, sit with your feet planted. Pull the heels towards your bottom and allow the pelvis to roll back. When only the tips of your toes touch the floor, grip your ankles with both hands and roll the upper body forward in a big arch. As you do so, pull the abdominal wall down and out and away from the thighs. For proper head alignment, keep your eyes on your heels or on the pelvis.

4.2.6 SINGLE-LEG STRETCH AND DOUBLE-LEG STRETCH

Goal: Strengthening the abdominal muscles and the core, improving coordination, improving trunk stability; learning about the relationship between the lower extremities and the core; promoting breath awareness.

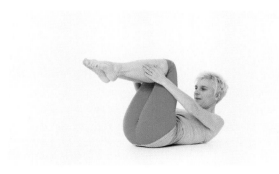

Starting position: On your back, the upper body is raised slightly (sternum drop); both legs are bent in a 90/90-degree position; hands rest on shins; the abdominal wall pulls deep, out, and up.

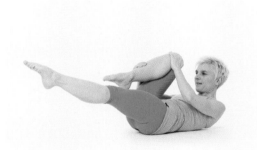

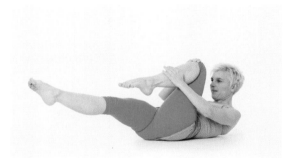

Execution: As you exhale, hold on to the bent right knee and make the left leg really long. At the same time, move the left hand to the right knee and the right hand below it to the shin or ankle, and pull the knee closer to the body. Hold for one breath, then switch sides. Both legs move at the same time and meet halfway. Hold the position again for one whole breath. Then make the movements more dynamic. As you inhale, extend the left leg and bend the right knee. As you exhale, extend the right leg and bend the left knee. Repeat 5-10x and switch legs (as you inhale, extend right, bend left, etc.).

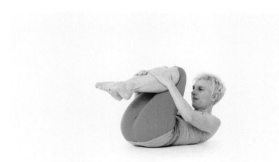

Variations: Change the breathing rhythm; begin with both hands at the chest; one foot on the floor; hands at the back of the head; place a ball or roller under the upper back.

For the double-leg stretch, pull your closed legs closer to the body as you exhale, while simultaneously pulling the abdominal wall in deep, wide, and long.

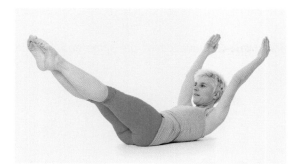
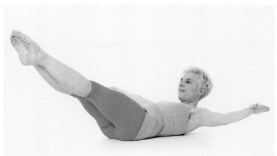

As you inhale, vigorously extend your closed legs while extending the arms overhead. Maintain your shoulder alignment and avoid arching the back. As you exhale, lower your arms to the sides and back down to your feet. When the arms are at shoulder level, bend your knees and return to the starting position. Feel how your movements support your breathing. Repeat the movement 5-10x.

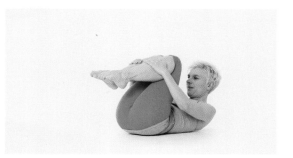

What to pay attention to: Your weight rests on your pelvis and ribcage; do not press your low back into the floor; lift the upper body to activate the upper abdominal muscles and make room for the lower abdomen (scoop); focus on controlling your midsection; maintain trunk alignment (no rotation); don't arch your back; keep the pelvis steady.

TIPS FOR PROS

When you extend a (both) leg(s) forward, also feel the pull in the hip joint and create the link between your lower extremities and the core. Lift the elbows to open the chest. Lift the head and shoulders far enough off the mat to feel your upper abdominals supporting them.

4.2.7 SPINAL STRETCH

Goal: Articulating the spine; opening up the low back; improving erection of the spine and posture; stretching the back of the legs; improving breathing.

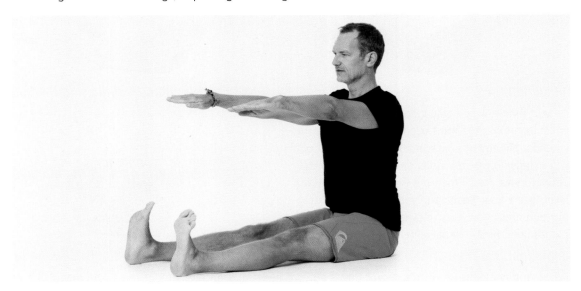

Starting position: In an upright seated position with legs extended and slightly more than hip-width apart; feet are flexed; gently press the heels into the floor; arms are extended forward at shoulder level in extension of the shoulders; fingers are long and palms face the floor.

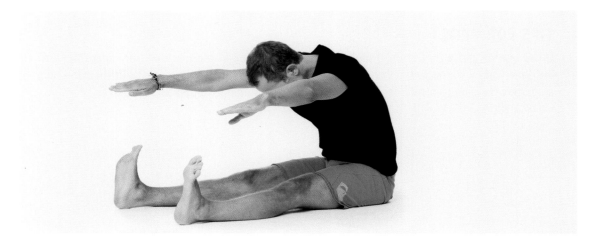

Execution: As you inhale, lengthen the spine, and actively push the sit bones into the floor as the crown of the head reaches up to the ceiling. As you exhale, begin to roll forward in a long uniform arch, starting with the head. As you do so, keep your sit bones firmly grounded and pull the abdominal wall in and up to create a counteraction. Push your arms forward as far as you can, parallel to the floor, without moving the pelvis. Doing so allows you to also stretch your low back. As you inhale, roll back to the upright seat, vertebrae by vertebrae. As you do so, actively push the sit bones into the floor and use your abdominal strength to come up. Repeat up to four times, going a little deeper each time.

What to pay attention to: Sit on your sit bones and actively lengthen the axis of the spine; allow the breath to flow slowly and evenly; kneecaps and toes point to the ceiling. Lengthen through your sit bones and the crown of the head before rolling forward in a big arch (don't let the head drop); your sit bones actively push into the mat during the entire movement; make sure the arch is uniform along the entire spine.

TIPS FOR PROS

Begin by pressing your hands into the mat between your legs to activate the abdominal muscles; imagine rolling over a big ball; your abdominal muscles roll your body forward, but simultaneously hold it up to ensure an even arch along the spine and to open your low back; use the breath to activate the abdominal muscles; imagine sitting against a wall and rolling up and down on it; focus on opening the low back; modify your seat or use aids to achieve neutral erection of the spine.

4.2.8 SAW

Goal: Articulating the spine; improving rotation; opening the low back; stretching the upper back; improving erection of the spine and posture; stretching the back of the legs; improving breathing; whittling the waist.

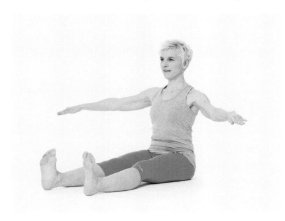

Starting position: Neutral seated position with legs extended and slightly more than hip-width apart; feet are flexed; arms are open to the sides at shoulder level in extension of the shoulder blades; palms face the floor and fingers are extended and touch.

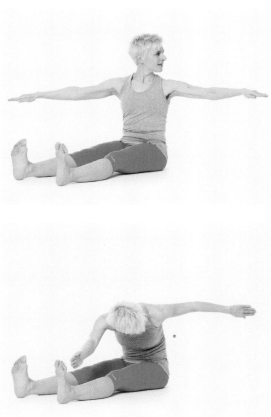

Execution: As you inhale, lengthen the spine, actively push the sit bones and heels into the floor, and rotate the upper body to the left. The upper body is erect, and the shoulders are parallel to the floor. As with the spinal twist, the arms reach out to the sides. As you exhale, roll your upper body forward. Your right pinkie reaches towards the left little toe. Your left arm reaches down and back, and internally rotates. The arms actively reach in opposite directions. Deepen the movement as though you were trying to listen to your left knee with your right ear. Your abdominal muscles lift the body and prevent you from "folding" over onto your leg. Your right pinkie wants to "saw" at the outside of your left little toe (three small pulses). As you inhale, vigorously push the sit bones into the mat and use your abdominal strength to roll back in the direction of rotation. As you exhale, deepen the twist before returning to the starting position. Repeat the movement 3x on each side.

What to pay attention to: Sit evenly on both sit bones and actively lengthen the axis of the spine; allow the breath to flow slowly and evenly; kneecaps and toes point to the ceiling; hold the head in extension of the spine during the entire movement sequence; the pelvis is neutral throughout; modify your seat or use aids to achieve a neutral erection of the spine.

TIPS FOR PROS

To learn this exercise, remain in each movement phase for a few moments to get a better feel for it; work with your feet against a wall to feel unintentional twisting of the pelvis or legs; begin by consciously moving into extension and rotation before rolling down.

4.2.9 SWAN DIVE

Goal: Activating the entire body; stabilizing the body in extension during a dynamic movement; strengthening all the muscles at the back of the body; massaging the internal organs.

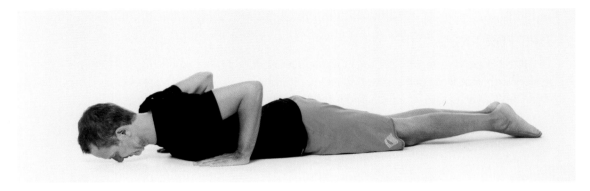

Starting position: On your stomach, legs are extended and closed; toes are pointed and hands are planted next to the ribcage; fingers are extended and palms are on the floor.

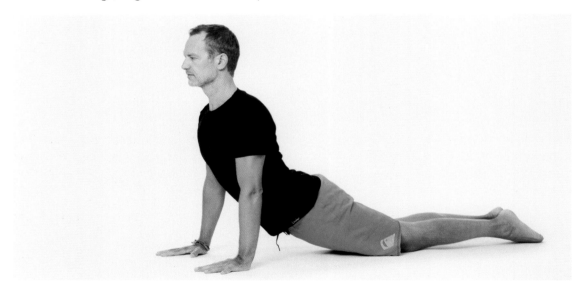

Execution: As you exhale, activate the core, lengthen the legs from the hips, lengthen the entire spine from the sacrum to the crown of the head, push the shoulder blades down towards the pelvis and lift the sternum. As you roll your upper body up off the mat in a long even arch, imagine pushing a small ball forward on the floor with your sternum. Vigorously press your hands into the floor and use your abdominal muscles to support the low back. When your arms are fully extended, widen the collar bones, inhale in preparation, and link the entire back of the body from the back of the head to the toes.

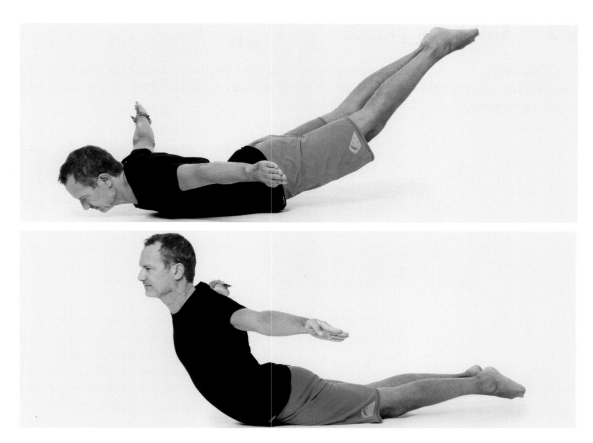

As you exhale, extend the arms to the sides and rock the body back and forth (like a rocking chair) 3x. Stabilize the rocker shape and keep your arms in lateral extension. After the third repetition, return your hands to starting position and catch your body in the lifted position. Inhale to lengthen the body further, and then start the next round as you exhale. Repeat this sequence up to 3x. After the final round, return to the supine position.

Variations: Easier: Elbows are bent; hands stay on the floor; practice with a ball under the pelvis. Harder: Don't put your hands on the floor; extend the arms next to your ears.

What to pay attention to: Keep the chest open and the back of the neck long. Keep the legs closed and maintain an even arch in the spine. Lengthen the body through the crown of the head. Avoid any pressure in the low back! Maintain axial extension and keep the abdominal muscles activated.

TIPS FOR PROS

Keep the elbows bent if your extension is not yet sufficient for a full backbend. Keep the hands on the mat for more control. Practice rocking the body on a stability ball by just bending and straightening the arms. Hold a Pilates ball between your ankles for more length. Hold a Pilates ball between your thighs to activate the adductor muscles more.

4.2.10 SHOULDER BRIDGE

Goal: Opening the front of the body from sternum to knees; stretching the hip flexors and back of the legs with a dynamic movement; strengthening the hip flexors and back of the legs with a dynamic movement; promoting abdominal strength and stability in extension.

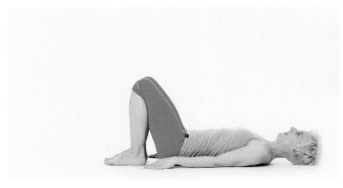

Starting position: On your back with knees bent; feet are planted below the knees in extension of the sit bones and legs are hip-width apart; arms are extended alongside the body with palms down.

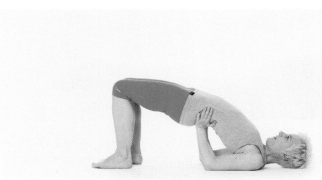

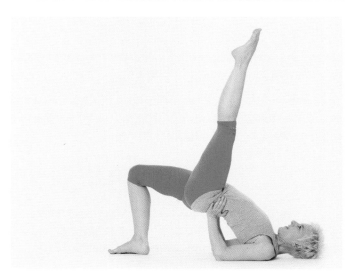

Execution: As you exhale, activate your core, vigorously press the feet into the floor, and flex the pelvis. As you continue to exhale, extend the knees towards the toes and roll the lower body up off the mat vertebrae by vertebrae. Lift the pelvis high enough so your elbows will be lined up with the shoulders and your hands can rest against the pelvis. The forearms are perpendicular to the floor and the fingertips point to the sides. Maintain a vigorous arch in the trunk and distribute your weight between the shoulder girdle, arms, and feet. Shift your weight to the right foot, and as you exhale, lift the left foot off the floor. Extend the left leg to the ceiling and vigorously push the right foot into the floor. As you exhale, point the foot and slowly lower the leg to the floor. As you do so, lengthen the leg from the hip and keep the rest of the body steady.

As you inhale, kick the leg up again. Repeat 3-5x, then bend the knee and move the leg back to starting position in the floor. Switch legs.

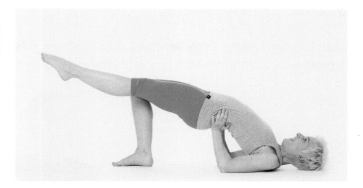

Variations: Keep the arms extended on the floor. The upper body forms a long line. Keep the knees bent and alternately lift them.

What to pay attention to: Maintain body alignment and keep the ribs integrated. Vigorously press the supporting foot into the floor and keep the supporting leg steady. Actively maintain the body's arch and don't rest the pelvis in your hands. Movement of the playing leg is controlled. No pressure on the nape! Don't arch the back!

TIPS FOR PROS

In case of discomfort in shoulders, elbows, or wrists, avoid using the arms for support. Flex the foot during the leg lift for a deeper stretch in the back of the legs. Gently lengthen the playing leg from the hip to open the hip more. Practice the movement with the pelvis on a ball or Pilates foam roller.

4.2.11 SPINAL TWIST

Goal: Improving rotation; strengthening the upper back; stretching the back and the back of the legs; improving respiration; improving erection of the spine and posture; whittling the waist.

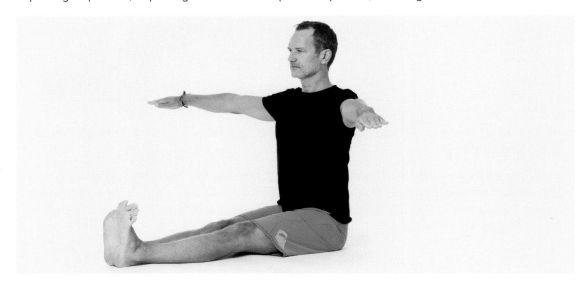

Starting position: Sit on the floor in an upright position with legs extended and closed; feet are flexed; gently press the heels into the floor; arms are laterally extended at shoulder level; fingers are long and palms face the floor.

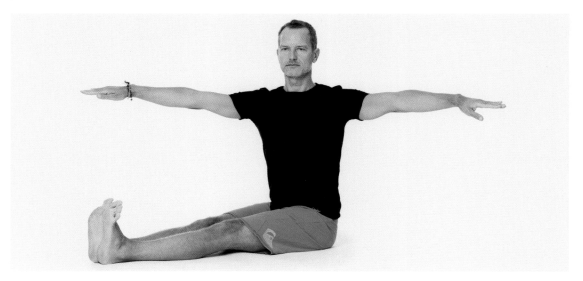

Execution: As you inhale, lengthen the spine, actively push the sit bones into the floor, and reach towards the ceiling with the crown of the head. Continue to lengthen the body and as you exhale, begin to twist the trunk to the left. Your head rotates with the spine and the gaze moves to the left. Feel your waist get longer and slimmer. As you inhale, return to the starting position. Repeat this sequence up to 4x, each time deepening the twist.

Variation: Sit with your legs in a moderate straddle to create a larger support surface; gently pulse 2-3x at the end of rotation.

What to pay attention to: Lengthen the spine as you twist; sit on your sit bones and actively lengthen the axis of the spine; allow the breath to flow slowly and evenly; kneecaps and toes point to the ceiling; rotate the trunk on the base of a steady pelvis; keep your bodyweight distributed evenly on your sit bones during the entire movement; keep your legs still on the floor; maintain alignment of arms, shoulders, neck, and head.

TIPS FOR PROS

Stabilize your seat with your heels and sit bones. If the back of the legs lack flexibility or there is a tendency to slump into the low back, bend the knees or cushion the pelvis. Bend the elbows and place the fingertips against the sternum to make sure you are moving your trunk and not just the arms. Begin practicing by placing your feet against a wall for a stable base. Imagine lengthening your arms from the sternum through the collarbones, the arms, hands, and fingers, all the way to the walls. Modify your seat or use aids to achieve neutral erection of the spine.

4.2.12 SIDE KICKS

Goal: Improving stability in a side-lying position; stretching the hip flexors and back of the legs with dynamic movements; strengthening the thigh and hip muscles.

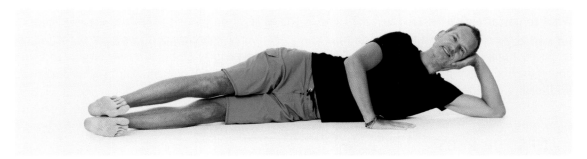

Starting position: On your side, place your bottom hand against the side of the head and lengthen the body via the elbow on the floor; keep the neck long and gently but deliberately press the head and hand together; rest your top hand palm down on the floor in front of your waist with the fingertips pointing towards the head; legs are extended and hips are slightly bent so your legs rest on the floor slightly in front of the body; the weight of the trunk rests on the pelvis and ribcage.

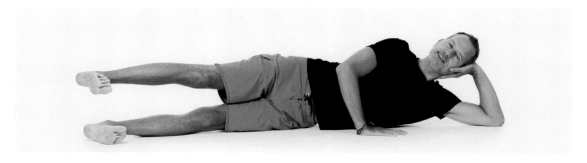

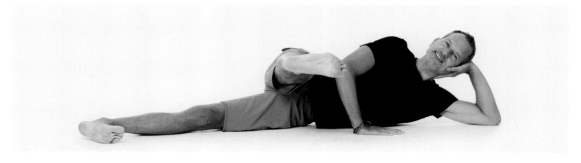

Execution: As you exhale, activate your core, lift the top leg, and extend it in extension of the body. As you inhale, swing the top leg forward parallel to the floor with the foot flexed until you feel a stretch in the back of the leg.

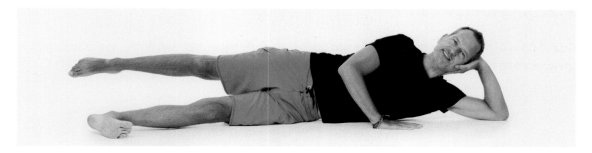

Lengthen the spine and keep the pelvis steady. Pulse once, then swing the leg back as you exhale until the hip is fully extended, pulse once, then start the movement over. Repeat 5-8x, then roll over on your stomach to the other side.

Variations: Lie on your extended bottom arm; rest on the forearm; rest both hands against the head; bend the bottom knee; bend the top knee; leg variations like cycling, leg circles, leg lifts. Very advanced: let the leg movement extend to the entire spine (lengthen the leg from the hip, flex the hip, flex the pelvis, flex the spine in an even arch, then extend the hip, extend the pelvis as well as the spine).

What to pay attention to: The top leg moves parallel to the floor to keep the upper body steady during the entire movement; keep the neck long and actively push the head and hand together; do not rest the head in the hand; lengthen the spine and legs as you swing the leg; isolate the leg movement; activate the core and gently push the lower half of the body into the floor; the weight of your trunk is distributed over the pelvis and ribcage.

TIPS FOR PROS

Start by practicing with your head on the floor and the bottom knee bent to achieve a stable side-lying position. Roll the pelvis back and forth a few times, then balance along the body's vertical axis for a neutral starting position. Place a towel between the bottom arm and the head for a long neck and good head alignment. Foot movement deepens the stretch, but requires more coordination.

4.2.13 TEASER

Goal: Maximum centering and control; articulating the spine; balancing; mobilizing and stabilizing the spine; working with axial extension and opposing forces; improving coordination.

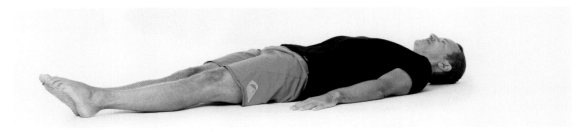

Starting position: On your back, legs are extended and closed; arms rest alongside the body palms down.

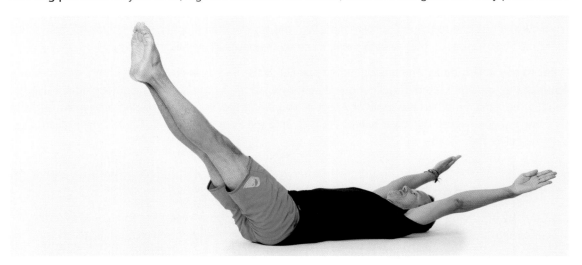

Execution: Teaser 1. Extend the arms overhead, bend the knees, move the knees over the hips and from there extend the legs towards the ceiling. Lower the legs to a 45-degree angle. Hold spine and pelvis in a neutral position and keep the core activated.

As you inhale, lift the extended arms so they are stacked over the shoulders. Fingertips point to the ceiling. As you exhale, roll up vertebrae by vertebrae starting with the head, and reach for your toes with your fingertips. Balance in this V-position for up to 3 breaths, lengthening through arms, legs, and the crown of the head. Keep the abdominal wall pulled in. As you exhale, roll back down to the floor very controlled while continuing to lengthen. When the head rests back on the floor, move the arms back overhead. Legs are still at a 45-degree angle. Repeat 3x, then bend the knees to relax.

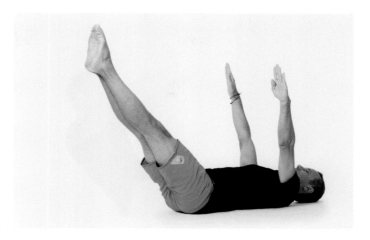

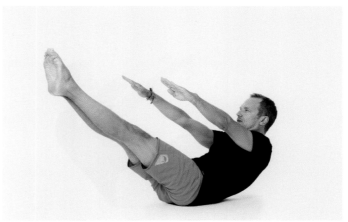

Or remain in a seated position and continue with teaser 2.

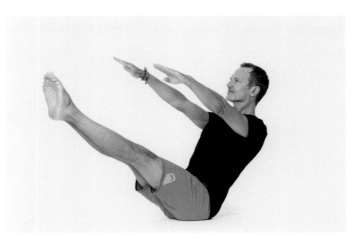

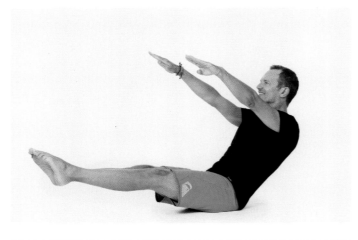

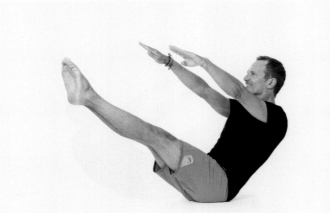

Teaser 2. Legs are raised at a 45-degree angle, the upper body is rolled up, and fingertips reach towards the toes. Keep the upper body completely quiet, and as you inhale, lower the legs as far as you can while still being able to control the movement. As you exhale, lift the legs again to a 45-degree angle. Repeat 3x, then roll back down to the floor in a controlled motion as you exhale, while continuing to lengthen. Legs and head arrive on the floor at the same time. As soon as the head rests on the floor, move the arms back to an overhead position and stretch the arms in the opposite direction of the legs. Then return to starting position.

Variations: Prepare for the teaser in a seated position with knees bent and small movements.

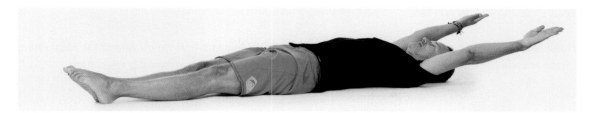

Teaser 3. Starting position as above with arms extended overhead. As you inhale, lift the arms towards the ceiling. As you exhale, simultaneously lift the extended legs and the head off the floor. Look at your toes and reach towards them with your fingertips until you are in a "V" position. As you exhale, roll back down on the floor. Head and legs arrive on the floor at the same time.

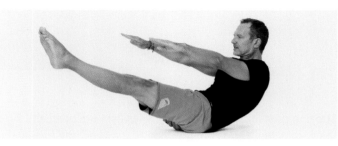

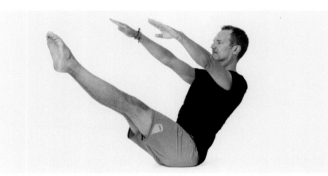

What to pay attention to: In teaser 1, hold the legs still and steady; keep the shoulder girdle organized; roll in a controlled motion without momentum; keep the legs extended and firmly closed; lengthen from the pelvis and don't slump; avoid breaking out to the sides while rolling; hold the head in extension of the spine; lengthen through arms and legs.

TIPS FOR PROS

Feel the connection between arms and back for good alignment of the shoulder girdle and head. Lengthen even the front of the body. Hold the legs of the person practicing or practice against a wall. Gently pull on the practicing person's arms or hands to support the rolling motion. Look in the desired direction of movement; create length in the body; use your abs and not your arms to roll up. Work with the flow of your breath without using momentum. Cushion the spine in places where your body doesn't touch the floor while rolling.

4.2.14 SWIMMING

Goal: Stabilizing the body in extension against opposing dynamic arm and leg movement; strengthening all the muscles at the back of the body; stretching the spine in extension; improving respiration.

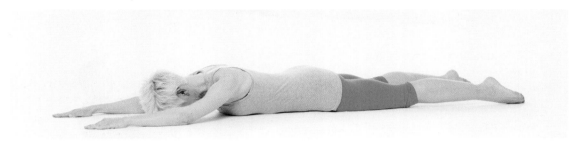

Starting position: On your stomach, legs are extended and hip-width apart; toes are pointed; arms rest on the floor palms down on either side of the head; the forehead rests on the floor.

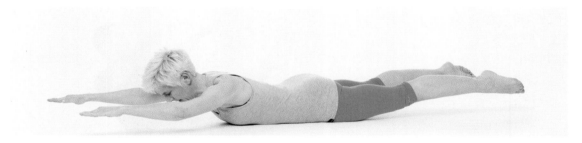

Execution: As you exhale, activate the core, lengthen the legs from the hips and the arms in the opposite direction; lengthen the entire spine from the tailbone to the top of the head; push the shoulder blades towards the pelvis and your sternum forward. As you peel your upper body off the floor in a long even arch, imagine pushing a small ball forward with your sternum. Support the low back with your abdominal muscles.

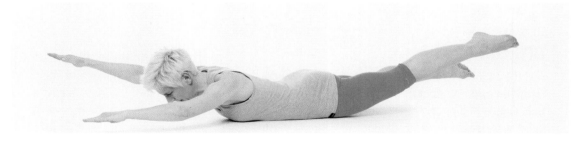

Next, lift the right arm and the left leg off the floor and continue to stretch them in opposite directions.

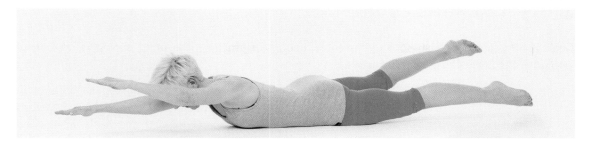

As you inhale, begin to swim by alternately lifting and lowering arms and legs on a diagonal. As you do so, inhale for 5 movements and exhale for 5 movements. Repeat several times, then return to starting position. From there, move into the child's pose position by sitting back on your heels. Actively keep the abdominal wall pulled in and up, and push your hands into the mat to stretch the back.

Variations: Swim with internal and external rotation; lengthen the breath.

What to pay attention to: Keep the abdominal wall activated; keep the chest open and the back of the neck long; support yourself with the strength of your entire back; keep the trunk steady while the arms and legs paddle vigorously; activate the gluteal muscles and the back of the legs; keep arms and legs extended; take slow, powerful breaths.

TIPS FOR PROS

To be more comfortable, place a towel under your forehead. Practice with a ball to lift the upper body if the shoulders cannot be sufficiently flexed. Begin by practicing extension of the hips and thoracic spine to take stress off the low back. Use the opposite arm and leg movement to stabilize the body during movement.

4.2.15 LEG PULL, FRONT

Goal: Strengthening and stabilizing the entire body, strengthening the arms, shoulders, and back; mobilizing the ankles; stretching the calves.

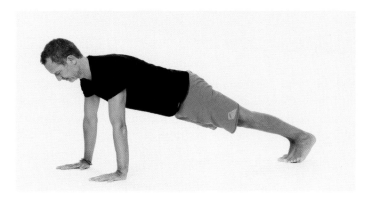

Starting position: In push-up position with hands below shoulders; fingertips point forward and heels are stacked over the balls of the feet; legs are closed and the head is an extension of the spine; actively push the hands into the floor.

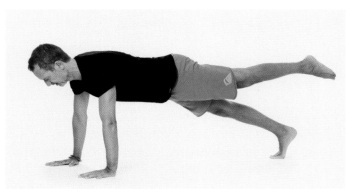

Execution: As you exhale, brush the left foot across the floor until it is fully extended and then raise the extended left leg.

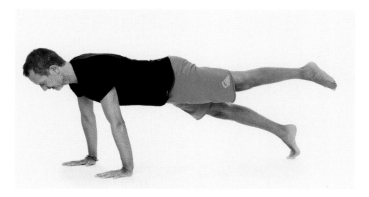

Reach way back with the left leg while pushing forward through the crown of the head and the right heel.

Keep pushing out through the crown of the head while pushing the right heel back. Then stack the right heel over the ball of the foot again and lengthen through the left heel as you return the left foot to starting position. With the next exhalation, repeat the movement sequence with the right leg. Repeat 3x per leg.

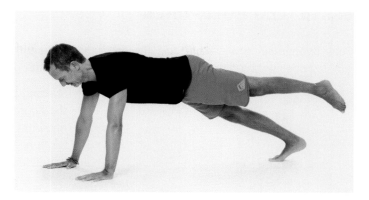

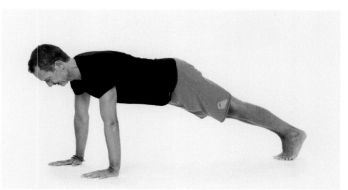

What to pay attention to: Maintain the space between the shoulder blades; firmly press the hands into the floor (wrist strength); fingertips face forward; extend elbows and knees without locking them; pelvis and low back remain neutral; keep the ribs integrated; hold the head in extension of the spine; lengthen the body between the soles of the feet and the crown of the head; raise the fully extended leg off the floor.

TIPS FOR PROS

Begin practicing by just raising and lowering the legs. Later, add the push forward, and after that do the entire sequence. In case of wrist problems, practice on your fists with palms facing inward, or with your forearms resting on a step.

4.2.16 LEG PULL, BACK

Goal: Strengthening and stabilizing the entire body; strengthening the arms, shoulders, and gluteal muscles; opening the chest and shoulders; stretching the back of the legs.

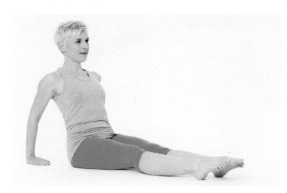

Starting position: Sit with your hands propped on the floor behind the hips; arms are extended and fingertips point forward; legs are extended and hip-width apart with the heels an extension of the sit bones; feet are gently pointed.

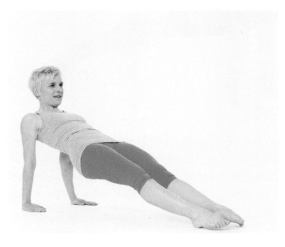

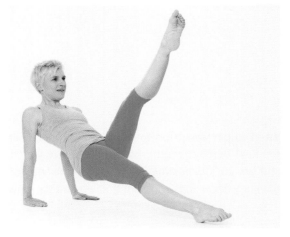

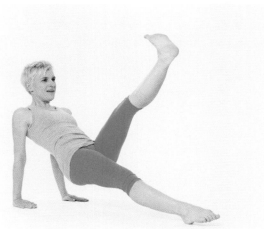

Execution: As you exhale, activate the core, actively press the hands and feet into the floor, fully extend the legs from the hips and lift the pelvis off the floor until the body forms a straight line. Look at your feet. Exhale and lift the left leg off the floor. Make as large a circle as possible with your toes. Flex the foot at the highest point of the movement to deepen the stretch in the back of the legs. As you inhale, lower the extended leg back down to the floor with the foot flexed. Push out vigorously through the heel. Switch sides. Repeat 3x per leg.

What to pay attention to: Maintain space between the shoulder blades and keep the neck long. Actively hold the head steady; it does not move forward or back. Firmly press the hands into the floor (wrist strength); fingertips point forward; straighten elbows and knees without locking them; pelvis and back remain neutral; keep the ribs integrated; lengthen the body between the soles of the feet and the crown of the head; lift the fully extended leg off the floor.

TIPS FOR PROS

Flex the feet for more stability in the trunk and knee of the supporting leg and a deeper stretch in the back of the moving leg. Lift the pelvis as you lower the leg. Support the pelvic lift with one hand under the practicing person's sacrum. Begin by practicing on the mat or sitting on a roller. In case of wrist pain, practice with the forearms resting on a step.

4.2.17 SIDE BEND

Goal: Strengthening and stabilizing in a side plank; promoting balance; strengthening arms and shoulders; strengthening and stretching the side of the body.

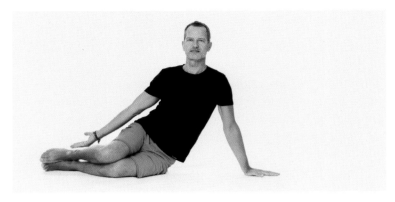

Starting position: Sit sideways on the left hip; knees are bent and stacked; the left hand is propped on the floor next to the left hip, and the left arm is extended and the fingers point to the left; the right hand rests on the right ankle. The soles of the feet, pelvis, trunk, and left hand are lined up.

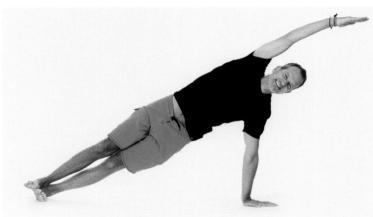

Execution: As you inhale, firmly press the outside edge of the left foot and the left hand into the floor. As you exhale, activate the core and lift the pelvis off the floor. The right arm sweeps up towards the ceiling and the body lengthens from the soles of the feet to the crown of the head.

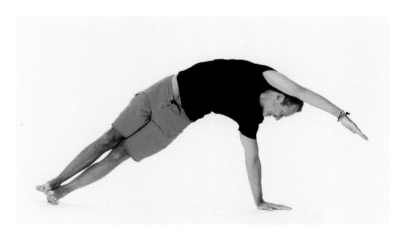

Still exhaling, continue to lengthen; lift the pelvis higher towards the ceiling while looking down at the floor next to your left hand.

As you inhale, move the right arm back to your right side, reach with your fingertips towards the feet, look down towards the feet and lower the pelvis towards the floor with legs extended. Repeat 2-3x, then bend the knees and return to starting position. Switch sides.

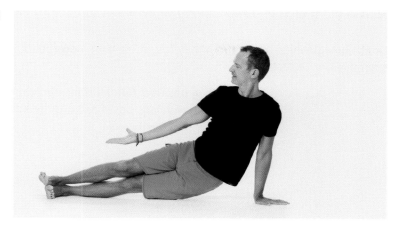

Variations: Bend the body towards the ceiling once, and then return to starting position.

What to pay attention to: Maintain the space between the shoulder blades; firmly press the hand into the floor; straighten the elbow without locking it; the pelvis remains in the frontal plane; keep the ribs integrated; lengthen the body between the soles of the feet and the crown of the head; breathe slowly and vigorously.

TIPS FOR PROS

Begin by placing the top foot under the bottom foot for better balance. The more the knees are bent in the beginning, the deeper is the side bend. Start by practicing with the knees just slightly bent. Practice the side bend towards the ceiling first. Later add the arching side bend. Do not do this exercise if you have pain in your wrists, elbows, or shoulders.

4.2.18 PUSH-UP

Goal: Strengthening the arms, shoulders, chest, and upper back; stretching the back of the legs; strengthening the core.

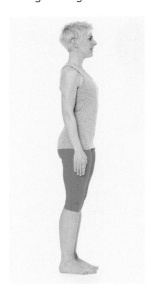

Starting position: Neutral stance with arms extended alongside the body (or standing with legs closed and slightly externally rotated; heels touching and toes slightly open).

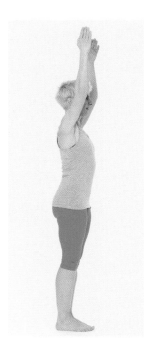

Execution: As you inhale, extend the arms to the ceiling and actively press the feet into the floor. As you exhale, activate the core, lower the arms to shoulder level and roll forward in an even arch until your hands touch the floor.

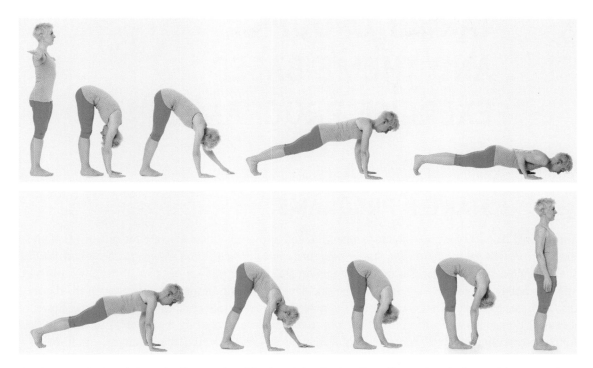

Firmly press the hands into the floor and pull in the abdominal wall. Walk your hands forward four steps into a push-up position. Hands are below shoulders and fingertips point forward. Legs are extended and heels are stacked over the balls of the feet. The body forms a long line from the top of the head to the soles of the feet. As you inhale, bend the elbows close to the side of the body while extending the body forward. As you exhale, straighten the arms. Walk your hands back four feet to your feet. As you do so, push the sit bones back and up. As you exhale, firmly press your hands and feet into the floor, then release the hands and roll vertebrae by vertebrae back up to an upright standing position and lift the arms overhead. Sweep the arms back down to your sides while reaching towards the ceiling with the top of your head. Repeat 3-4x.

Variations: Lateral arm extension; more push-ups per set; lift the heels; on one leg.

What to pay attention to: Maintain the space between the shoulder blades and the head as an extension of the spine; keep the abdominal wall engaged; lumbar spine and pelvis remain neutral and ribs are integrated; hands are directly below the shoulders and fingertips point forward; elbows are straight but not locked; elbows touch the ribcage while bending.

TIPS FOR PROS

· In case of wrist pain, work on your fists with palms facing inward. Rest one hand on the crown of the head to feel the head reaching forward. Fix the heels or rest the feet against a wall during the push-up movement. First practice the individual elements, and then combine them into a series.

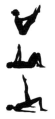

5 TARGET GROUPS AND THEME-BASED EXERCISE PROGRAMS

5.1 STARTER PROGRAMS

They should be part of every instructor's repertoire and at the same time they are the greatest challenge: exercise concepts for beginners. Our starter programs can be completed on the spot as described. Each of the movement sequences focuses on just one motor skill or principle. For instance, if the emphasis is on strength ability, the exercise is easy or rather one-dimensional with respect to coordination (by the way, also a Pilates principle). That is the case if the movement takes place on only one plane and is slower or steady. If the emphasis is on coordination, less strength effort is required. It also helps to teach in flow form (also an original Pilates concept). That means the exercises flow together seamlessly. That makes it easier for the participant to focus (concentration is another original Pilates principal). The challenge in designing a beginner program lies in combining exercises that are easy to execute but are also exciting, and in making it easy to learn and internalize the Pilates principles.

TIPS FOR INSTRUCTORS

Familiarize your participants with the centering and breathing exercises at the beginning of the unit (see pages 19-41). This will help them better execute the individual exercises. You can repeat the series over a period of several weeks. When changing the order of the exercises, make sure the transitions are calm and focused, in a flow. Verbal instructions should go from general to detailed: begin with the movement description, explain the beginning, progression, and end of the exercise, add the breathing rhythm, then the primary principle you are working on. This allows the participants to perform the exercises accurately.

TIP FOR STUDENTS

Use your breath to set the rhythm. It will allow you to practice with lots of focus and you will feel precisely which pace the exercise requires. This can be quite unfamiliar at first, but will gradually become more natural.

5.1.1   STARTER PROGRAM 1

LOW ABS

Starting position: Neutral supine position with knees bent and feet planted. Legs are parallel and hip-width apart. Arms rest alongside the body.

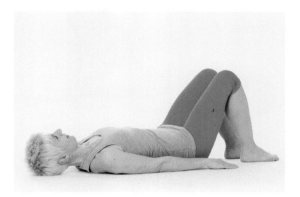

Execution: As you exhale, pull the knees towards the body one at a time until hips and knees are at a 90-degree angle. Take a breath, and with the next exhalation place the feet back on the floor one at a time. Alternate starting with the left and the right leg.

Repeat 4-5x on each side.

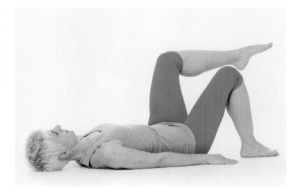

IMPORTANT
The pelvis remains steady on the floor even when the second leg is lifted.

BASIC BRIDGE

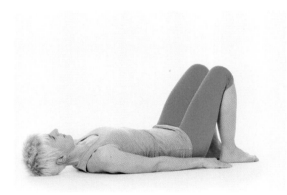

Starting position: Neutral supine position with knees bent and feet planted. Heels are below the knees; legs are parallel and hip-width apart; arms rest alongside the body.

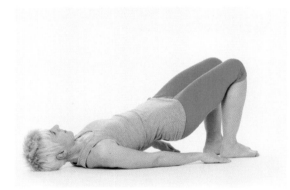

Execution: As you exhale, roll the spine up from the tailbone to the shoulder girdle.

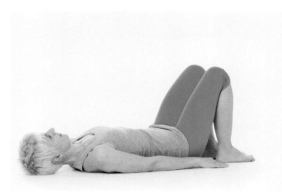

Take a breath, and with your next exhalation roll back down vertebrae by vertebrae to the starting position.

Repeat 6-8x.

IMPORTANT

Only roll up as far as the shoulder girdle, meaning up to the shoulder blades. The cervical spine remains long.

STERNUM DROP

Starting position: Neutral supine position with knees bent and feet planted. Legs are parallel and hip-width apart; arms rest alongside the body.

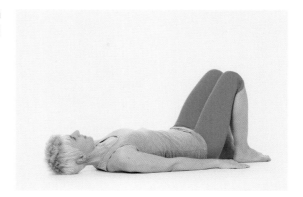

Execution: As you exhale, reach with your hands towards your feet and roll up head and shoulders to the shoulder girdle.

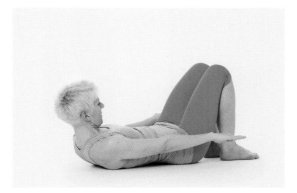

As you inhale, roll back down vertebrae by vertebrae to the starting position.

Repeat 6-8x.

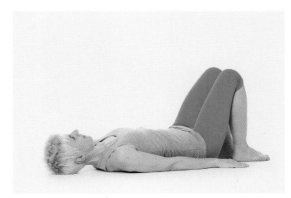

TIP

The gaze is directed at the thighs. This results in an economical execution of the exercise because it facilitates the ventral connection and takes stress off the cervical spine and the shoulder and nape area.

SINGLE-LEG STRETCH

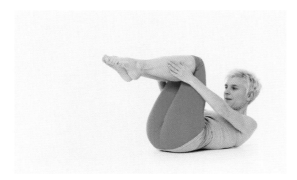

Starting position: On your back; head and shoulder girdle are rolled up (sternum drop); legs are in a 90/90-degree position; hands rest on shins.

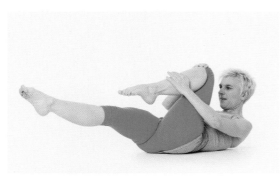

Execution: Working with your breath, extend one leg at a time while holding on to the bent knee with your hands.

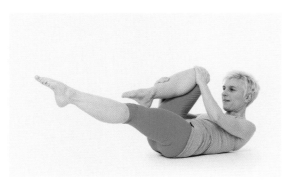

Switch legs as you exhale.

Repeat 4-6x per side.

IMPORTANT
The trunk remains stable when the legs change position.

TWIST

Starting position: Sitting in a cross-legged position, arms are laterally extended at shoulder level.

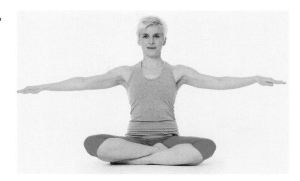

Execution: As you exhale, rotate the spine around its vertical axis; the gaze moves in the direction of rotation.

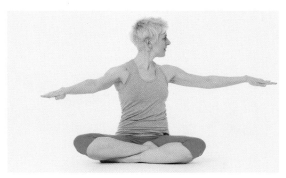

As you inhale, return to the starting position.

Repeat 4-6x per side.

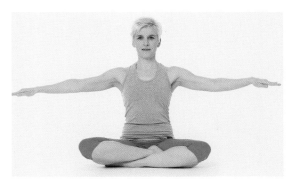

IMPORTANT

The movement originates from the rotation of the trunk and not hyperextension of the shoulders. Maintain alignment of the arms relative to the shoulder girdle.

HIP STRETCH

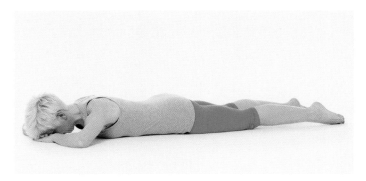

Starting position: On your stomach, the forehead rests on the back of the hands.

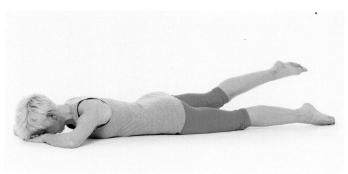

Execution: As you exhale, slightly lift the right leg off the floor from the hip.

As you inhale, lower the leg back to the floor.

Repeat 6-8x, alternating sides.

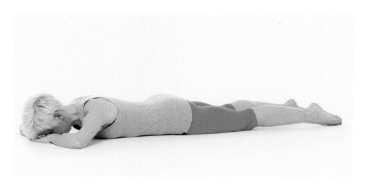

IMPORTANT
Stay centered.

MAD CAT

Starting position: On all fours.

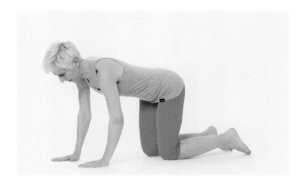

Execution: As you exhale, press your hands and legs into the floor and round the spine.

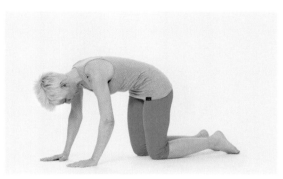

As you inhale, return to the starting position.

Repeat 6-8x.

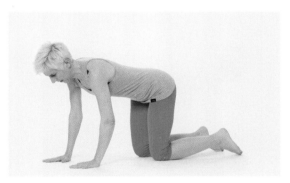

IMPORTANT

To round the lumbar spine, pull the abdominal wall in.

UP STRETCH

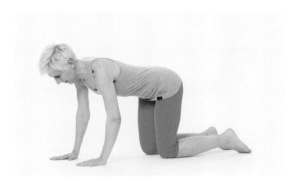

Starting position: On all fours.

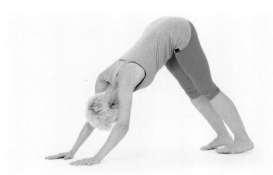

Execution: As you exhale, straighten the legs and lift the pelvis towards the ceiling.

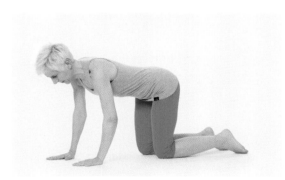

As you inhale, return to the starting position.

Repeat 6-8x.

IMPORTANT

Push your sit bones up towards the ceiling while pushing the heels towards the floor.

RELAXATION

Starting position: Child's pose with arms alongside the body.

Execution: Take several breaths to relax the back and allow the upper body to sink deeper against the thighs.

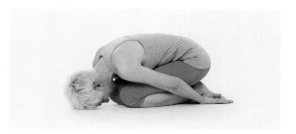

TIP

Purposefully send the inhaled breath to different sections of the spine (e.g., lumbar spine or thoracic spine).

ALL OF THE EXERCISES AT A GLANCE

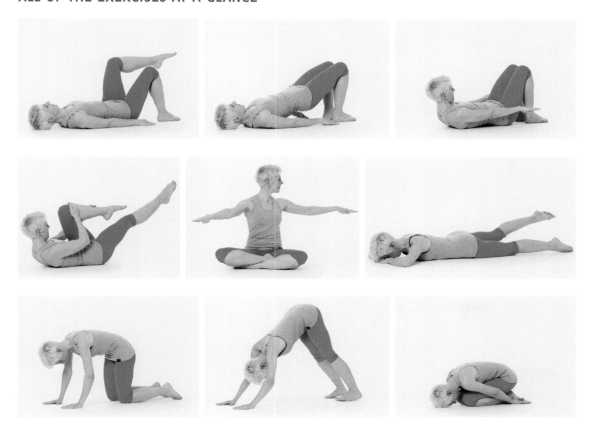

5.1.2   STARTER PROGRAM 2

FLOATING ARMS

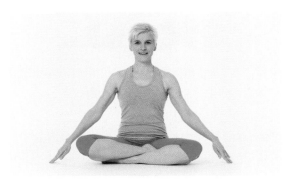

Starting position: Cross-legged seat, arms are relaxed at the sides.

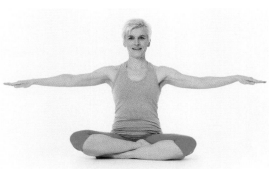

Execution: As you exhale, drag the fingertips sideways along the floor, and from there, lengthen the arms and allow them to pull up to shoulder level.

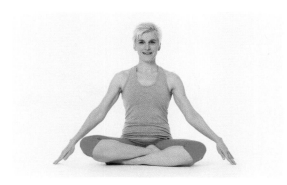

As you inhale, lower the arms.

Repeat 6-8x.

IMPORTANT

The shoulder blades slide first towards the pelvis via the rear costal arches, then to the spine, and then to the outside.

SIDE BEND

Starting position: Cross-legged seat, arms rest at the sides, palms face the floor.

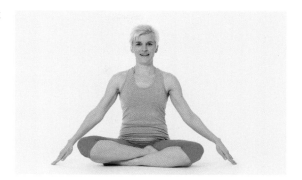

Execution: As you inhale, lift the spine. As you exhale, reach with your right arm first to the side and then sweep it up and over your head to the opposite side. The spine bends sideways in a big arch, the left elbow is bent and the right hand lightly rests on the floor for support.

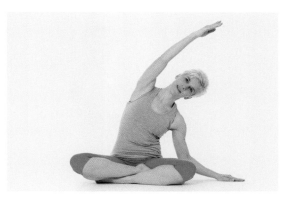

As you inhale, return to the starting position.

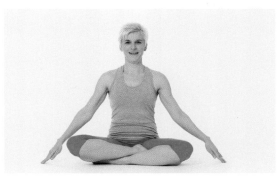

IMPORTANT

Both sit bones maintain contact with the floor; all of the movement takes place on the frontal plane.

HALF ROLL BACK

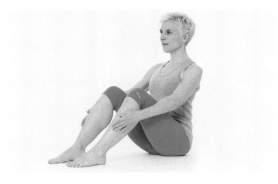

Starting position: Neutral seated position; feet at planted and hip-width apart; hands grip the knees.

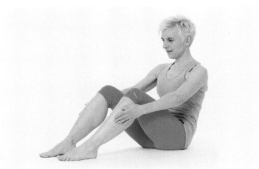

Execution: As you inhale, lift the spine and push the top of the head towards the ceiling. As you exhale, pull the abdominal wall in, and tilt the pelvis back until the spine forms a "C" shape. The gaze is forward and down, and the arms are extended.

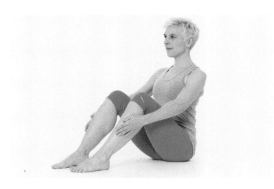

As you inhale, return to the starting position beginning with the head.

IMPORTANT

The spine's "C" shape is even and the shoulder girdle remains wide open.

STERNUM DROP

Starting position: On your back, feet are planted; hands are folded behind the head.

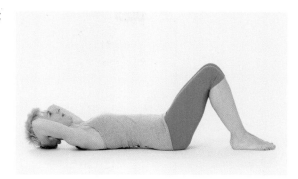

Execution: As you exhale, roll head and shoulders up while looking towards the abdominal wall.

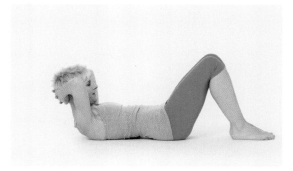

As you inhale, return to the starting position.

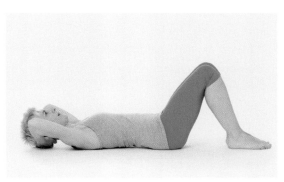

PLEASE NOTE
The head is cradled in the hands; do not pull up with the elbows.

ONE HUNDRED

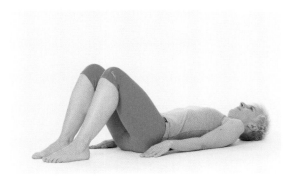

Starting position: On your back, knees are bent, and feet are planted; arms rest alongside the body palms down.

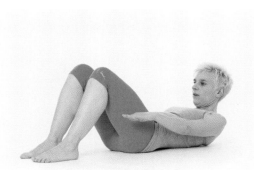

Execution: Begin by rolling up head and shoulders. Then take 5 short breaths through the nose and exhale 5x through the nose or mouth. As you do so, vigorously pump the arms up and down. Pump up to 100x, then roll head, arms, and legs back down to the mat.

TIP
Gradually increase the breaths: first inhale 2x and exhale 2x; then 3x, 4x, etc.

SIDE KICK PREPARATION

Starting position: On your side, the bottom arm is extended; the hand of the top arm rests on the floor in front of the sternum and stabilizes the side-lying posture; legs and hips are bent 90 degrees; the back of the head, thoracic spine, and sacrum are lined up along the back edge of the mat or along an imaginary line; the top leg is raised to hip level.

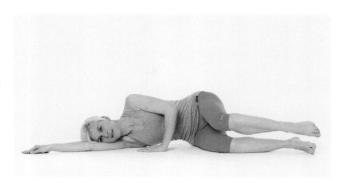

Execution: As you inhale, flex the hip and move the knee forward.

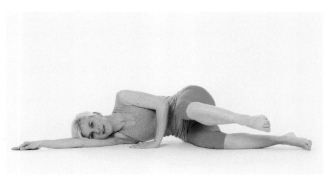

As you exhale, extend the hip and move the top leg back.

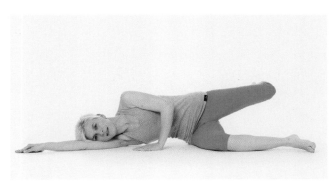

IMPORTANT

The pelvis remains steady. Think about the air cushion below the waist.

COBRA

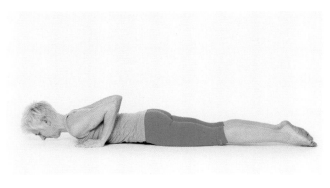

Starting position: On your stomach, hands are propped below the shoulders (acromion).

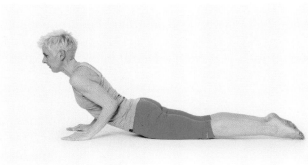

Execution: As you exhale, press the hands into the floor; elbows pull towards the feet, the sternum pushes forward, and the spine lengthens.

With the next exhalation, reverse the sequence to return to the start.

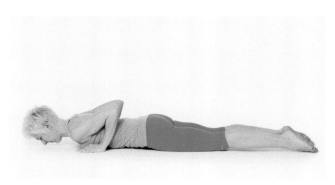

IMPORTANT

Stay centered to stabilize the lumbar spine.

STRETCHING DOG

Starting position: On all fours.

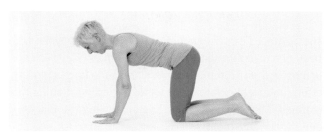

Execution: As you exhale, shift your weight to the right hand and left leg, and first drag the left arm and right leg along the floor, before lifting both off the floor in full extension.

Repeat and alternate sides 4-6x.

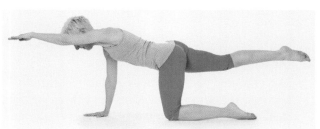

IMPORTANT
Every arm and leg movement is preceded by a shift in bodyweight.

ALL OF THE EXERCISES AT A GLANCE

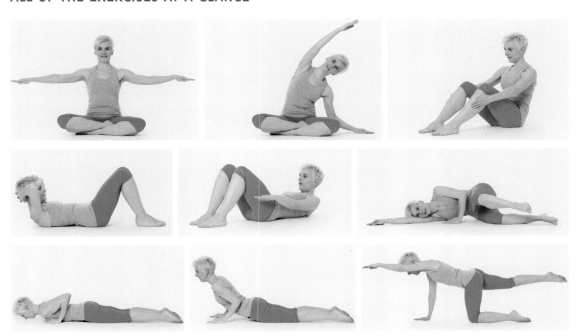

5.2 EXERCISE PROGRAMS FOR ADVANCED STUDENTS

The advanced exercise programs are geared to anyone with previous Pilates experience or those who have been practicing for some time with our book. The method's principles as well as basic motor skills must be understood and internalized. Now it is time for students to be guided to the next level. It requires greater effort, and axial extension becomes the foundation for mastering the exercises. More coordination is also required. Movements become spatial, linking the planes of movement of the basic exercises. The rhythm gets faster and breathing in support of exercise execution becomes increasingly important. Complete focus (concentration) is now necessary to enjoy the flow of the exercises.

TIPS FOR INSTRUCTORS

Even advanced participants need a moment to settle in, get focused, and prepare the body for the exercises. The advanced exercises can only be mastered safely with good preparation and a solid build-up. Find a common thread in the exercises and carefully increase the degree of difficulty. Your instructions can now deepen understanding of the exercises, but should not overwhelm the participant with information. The right amount of information is important for the class flow and dynamics. With experienced participants that have mastered the exercises, you can increasingly emphasize the rhythm and dynamics, and only offer detailed information as needed. Never forget that the participant's safety and well-being are a priority and must never be sacrificed in favor of a fancy exercise sequence. Avoid using the class as a stage and keep your focus on all participants.

TIPS FOR STUDENTS

Internalize the movement sequences and memorize the exercise sequence. This will allow you to fully focus on the flow of exercises. Create a place where you can practice undisturbed and find a ritual that allows you to focus completely on yourself and your practice. If you wish to practice longer, do not increase the number of repetitions, rather supplement your program with exercises from our exercise catalogue.

If you are unsure about the execution of the exercises, get help from a competent Pilates instructor in your area. The major training facilities as well as some sporting goods suppliers will have the names of reputable instructors and will gladly help you in your search.

5.2.1 PROGRAM 1 FOR ADVANCED STUDENTS

Start by taking a few breaths while lying on your back to get in the right mindset. Find your neutral supine position, and build up your Pilates breathing and get centered. Begin by fully focusing on the exercises.

ROLL UP

Starting position: On your back with legs extended; arms rest alongside the body.

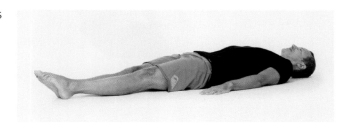

Execution: As you inhale, lift the arms so they are stacked over the shoulders; as you exhale, roll up vertebrae by vertebrae starting with the head all the way to the sit bones until the upper body is extended over the legs in a long even arch.

With your next inhalation, start to roll back down vertebrae by vertebrae, exhale and continue to roll down, and as soon as your head touches the floor lift the arms towards the head.

Repeat 3-4x.

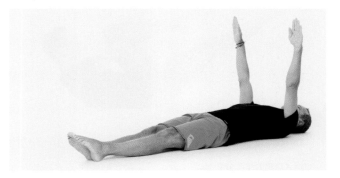

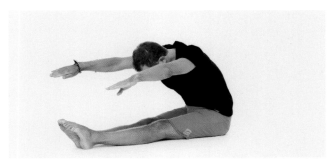

TIP

Look in the direction of movement; if necessary, cushion the spine.

SINGLE-LEG STRETCH

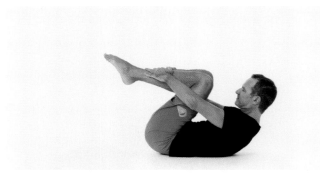

Starting position: On your back, the upper body is rolled up to the shoulder blades (sternum drop); both knees are bent in the air and hands grip the lower legs.

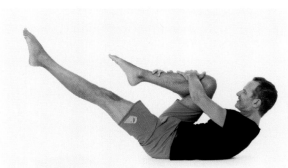

Execution: As you exhale, extend the left leg forward and hold on to the right leg with your hands. As you inhale, start to extend the right leg and bend the left knee. The legs meet halfway. As you exhale, extend the right leg and hold the lower left leg with both hands.

Repeat 3-5x per leg.

IMPORTANT

Hold the upper body steady. Legs are extended at approximately a 45-degree angle. Move rhythmically and evenly.

CRISS-CROSS

Starting position: On your back, the upper body is rolled up to the shoulder blades (sternum drop); both knees are bent in the air; hands are folded at the back of the head.

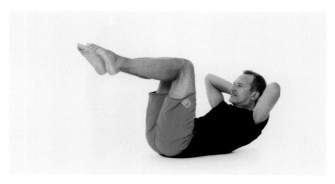

Execution: As you exhale, extend the right leg forward and pull the left elbow back. As you inhale, return to the starting position. With the next exhalation, start the same movement on the other side.

Repeat 3-5x per leg.

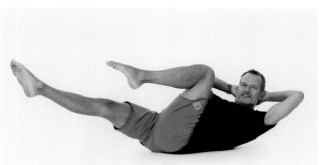

TIP

Turn your head and gaze in the direction of the elbow that rolls back. Focus on the extension part of the movement and not the convergence of elbow and knee.

IMPORTANT

The hands support the head like a hammock. The pelvis is steady. Legs are extended forward at approximately a 45-degree angle. Move rhythmically and evenly, like the single-leg stretch with the added rotation of the trunk!

SPINAL STRETCH

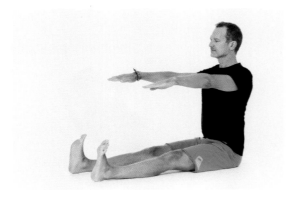

Starting position: Sit with your legs extended; legs are shoulder-width apart and arms are extended forward parallel, at shoulder level.

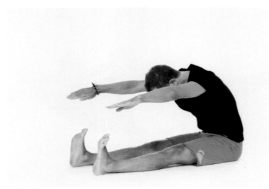

Execution: As you exhale, roll forward vertebrae by vertebrae starting with the head. Arms remain parallel to the floor and the head stays higher than the arms. As you inhale, roll back to your upright seat.

TIP

Imagine you are sitting against a wall—or actually sit against a wall. Peel off the wall to roll forward, and then roll back up against the wall. Look in the direction of movement.

SAW

Starting position: Sit with your legs extended; legs are mat-width or slightly further apart; arms are extended laterally at shoulder level, palms face down.

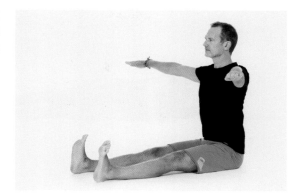

Execution: As you inhale, lengthen the body and twist to the left. As you do so, the right arm externally rotates and the left arm internally rotates. As you exhale, roll forward vertebrae by vertebrae starting with the head. As you do so, reach for the left little toe with your right pinkie. As you inhale, roll back up to your upright seat, then exhale and turn to the right to return to the starting position.

Repeat 3x per side.

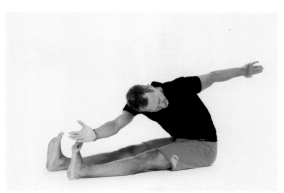

TIP

Anchor yourself with your heels and sit bones, and make sure that anchor remains stable. Turn your head as though you were trying to listen closely to your knee. Rotate the palms forward to create more space in the shoulders. Bend the knees or raise your seat if necessary.

SIDE-LYING DOUBLE-LEG LIFT, RIGHT

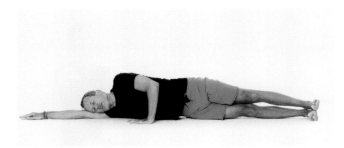

Starting position: Lie on your right side with the head resting on the extended right arm; the palm faces the floor and the left arm is propped on the floor in front of the ribcage for support.

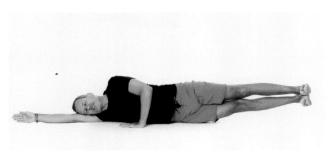

Execution: As you exhale, activate the core and the adductors and slightly lift your closed legs of the floor. As you inhale, lower the legs back to the starting position.

Repeat 5-8x.

After some practice, also extend the right arm on the floor and lift the upper body along with the legs.

Repeat 3x.

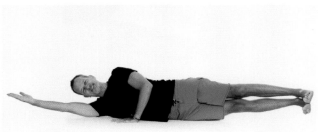

TIP
Imagine lying against a wall with the back of your head, ribcage, pelvis, and heels touching the wall. Use a pillow if you lack the shoulder mobility to rest your head on the extended lower arm. Place a rolled-up towel under the waist to create more length.

SIDE-LYING DOUBLE-LEG LIFT, LEFT

See side-lying double leg-lift, right.

SWAN DIVE 1

Starting position: On your stomach with legs extended; hands are planted next to the ribcage.

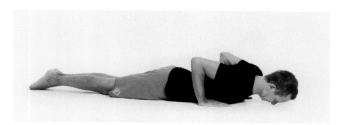

Execution: As you exhale, lift the upper body off the floor in a long arch.

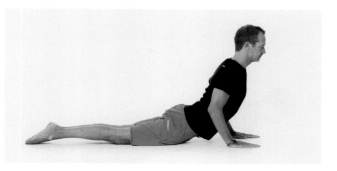

Lengthen the body as you inhale and create a powerful line from the soles of the feet to the back of the head. As you exhale, start to lower the upper body while simultaneously lifting the legs off the floor. As you inhale, reverse the motion sequence. Keep your hands next to you on the mat throughout the exercise.

Repeat 3-5x, then move into child's pose.

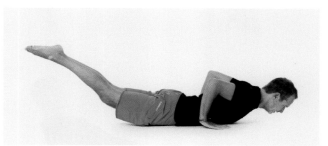

TIP
Imagine you are moving like the rocker of a rocking horse.

IMPORTANT
Mastering this exercise requires good extension of the thoracic spine and hips. Start with the elbows bent to take the stress off the lumbar spine. Keep the body long and centered! To take stress off the back of the neck, look for the perceived feeling of the sternum being higher than the head.

CONTROL FRONT, CONTROL BACK

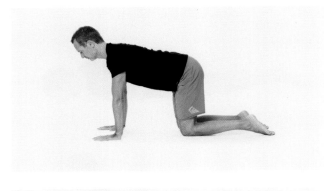

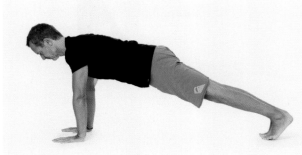

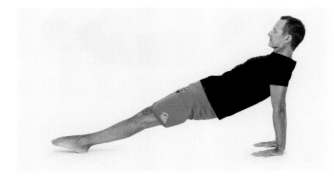

Starting position: Neutral all-fours position.

Execution: As you exhale, extend the legs back one at a time, assuming a push-up position. Hold for one inhalation. As you exhale, return to the all-fours position. Start the next set with the other leg.

Repeat 4x.

To do the control back exercise, move the right foot to the left hand and cross the left leg behind it from the last push-up position, and then return via the cross-legged position to a seated posture with legs extended forward.

Prop your hands behind your hips with fingers pointing forward. As you inhale, create space between the shoulders, activate the core and firmly press the hands into the floor. As you exhale, lift the pelvis off the floor. Hold for one inhalation, and as you exhale, lower the pelvis back down in a controlled motion.

Repeat 3-4 x.

IMPORTANT

The pelvis is stable. The spine is neutral. Maintain length. Elbows are soft. Shoulders are in proper alignment!

ROLLING BACK

Starting position: Sit with your knees bent and feet planted; hands grip the shins; the upper body forms a perfect arch from the tailbone to the top of the head.

Execution: As you exhale, pull the heels close to your bottom and balance on your sacrum. As you inhale, roll back to the shoulder girdle. As you exhale, roll back up into your balancing pose.

Repeat 6-8x. With the final rolling motion, move into a squat or come directly to a standing pose for the push-up series.

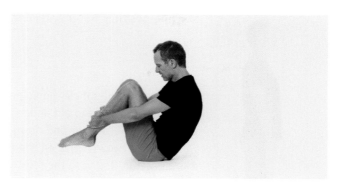

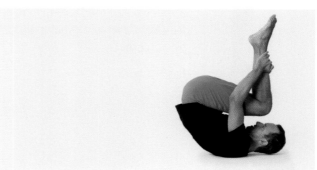

IMPORTANT

Actively pull the abdominal wall away from the thighs. Maintain the ball shape throughout the entire motion sequence. Do not use momentum from the legs, and don't roll onto the head.

PUSH-UP SERIES

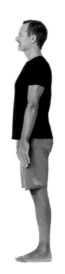

Starting position: Neutral standing pose.

Execution: As you inhale, firmly press your feet into the floor while reaching for the ceiling with the top of the head. Create axial length and activate the core. As you exhale, roll forward and down in an even arch starting with the head, until you can plant your hands on the floor. Walk your hands forward three steps in a straight line, and with the fourth step move into a push-up position. Bend the elbows 1-3x as you exhale and straighten them as you inhale. Then move into an up stretch (see the Starter Programs) as you exhale. Walk your hands back to your feet. With the next exhalation, roll back up into the starting position vertebrae by vertebrae.

Repeat 1-3 x.

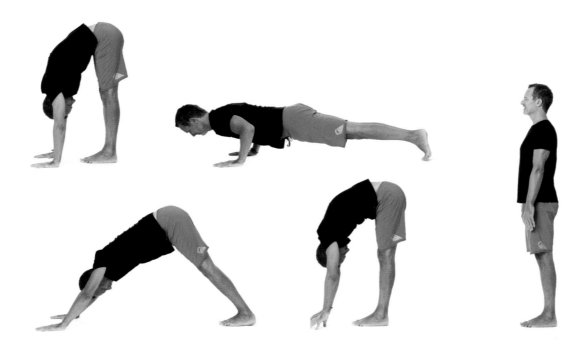

TIP

To master the exercise, look for axial extension throughout the exercise. Bend the knees if you don't have sufficient flexibility or strength.

End the exercise sequence by taking several breaths in the standing position to rest and reflect.

ALL OF THE EXERCISES AT A GLANCE

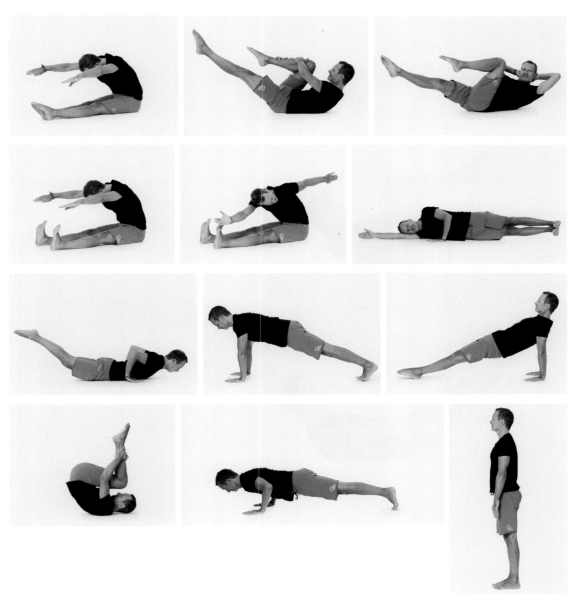

PILATES

5.2.2 PROGRAM 2 FOR ADVANCED STUDENTS

Begin by doing some circling motions over your feet in a standing position to find proper foot alignment. Lengthen your horizontal axis of shoulder girdle and hips as well as the vertical axis of your spine. Begin Pilates breathing and activate the core.

Now roll forward vertebrae by vertebrae in the biggest arch possible until your fingertips touch the floor. Move into a squat and then onto your back for the one hundred.

Important: Actively press the feet into the floor for more axial length. The abdominal wall stays engaged. Keep the pelvis over the feet. Roll evenly along the spine and bend the knees if necessary. Allow the head to hang loosely.

ONE HUNDRED

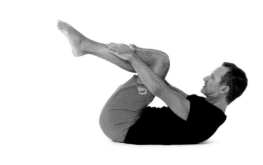

Starting position: On your back, head and shoulders are rolled up; knees are lifted and closed; hold the knees above the hips; knees are bent approximately 90 degrees; hands rest on the lower legs.

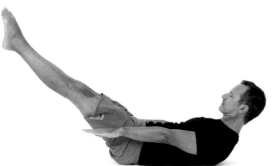

Execution: As you exhale, reach with your hands towards your feet while extending the legs.

As you exhale, start pumping the arms vigorously up and down. Pump 5x per inhalation and exhalation.

Repeat up to 10x.

DOUBLE-LEG STRETCH

Starting position: On your back; roll the upper body up to the shoulder blades (sternum drop); both knees are bent in the air and hands rest on the shins.

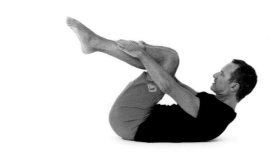

Execution: As you exhale, extend the closed legs forward at a 45-degree angle and extend the parallel arms towards the head at the same angle. As you inhale, circle the arms to the outside; when the arms are at approximately shoulder level, bend the knees and return to the starting position.

Repeat 3-5x.

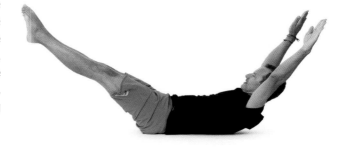

IMPORTANT
The upper body remains steady. Move rhythmically and evenly.

SPINAL TWIST

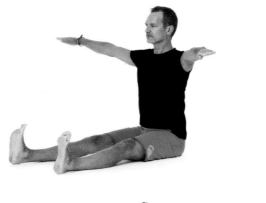

Starting position: Neutral seat with legs extended; legs are shoulder-width apart; arms are laterally extended at shoulder level, palms down.

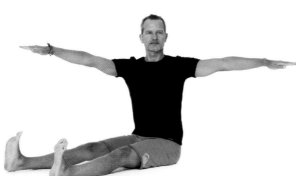

Execution: As you inhale, lengthen the body and as you exhale, twist to the left; as you inhale, return to the starting position. Repeat 3x per side.

Variation: Legs closed; three little pulses at the end of rotation.

TIP

Anchor yourself with your heels and sit bones and make sure that anchor remains stable. Turn your palms forward to create more space in the shoulders; imagine yourself doing a spiraling movement towards the ceiling.

SIDE KICK SERIES, RIGHT

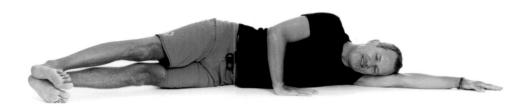

Starting position: Neutral side-lying position with the head resting on the extended left arm; the palm faces the floor and the right arm is propped in front of the ribcage for support; Legs are closed and a slight forward angle to the body.

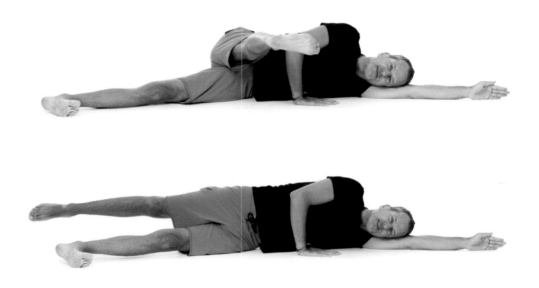

Execution: As you exhale, lengthen the body from the tailbone to the top of the head; activate the core and lift the right leg so it hovers parallel to the mat. As you inhale, flex the hip and move the extended right leg forward. As you exhale, extend the hip and move the extended right leg back. Repeat 3-5x.

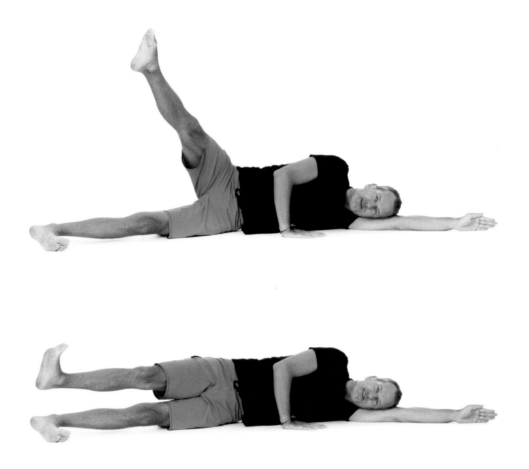

Move the right leg back to the starting position and externally rotate it. Lift the leg as you inhale and lower the leg against resistance as you exhale. Repeat 3-5x.

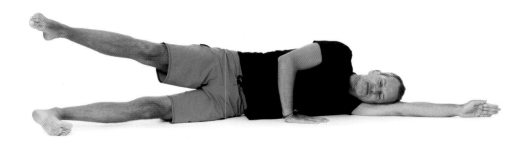

Next describe small circles with the top leg, 3-5x in each direction.

Make the movements only as big as you can control.

TIP

Imagine lying with your body against a wall and the back of your head, the ribcage, and the pelvis are touching the wall. For more stability, move the extended bottom leg forward slightly on the floor or bend it.

IMPORTANT

The weight of the trunk is distributed between the pelvis and the ribcage, not in between. Use a pillow if a lack of shoulder mobility won't allow you to rest your head on the extended arm. Place a rolled-up towel under the waist for more length. Keep the body long and centered!

SIDE KICK SERIES, LEFT

See side kick series, right.

SWIMMING

Starting position: On your stomach with arms and legs extended; arms are on either side of the head.

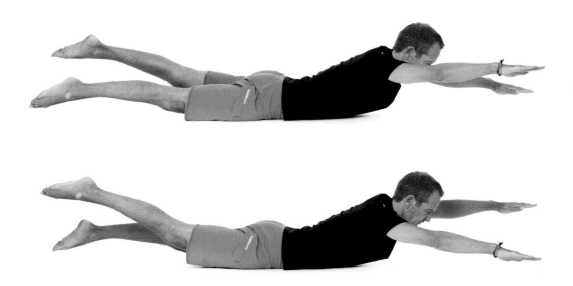

Execution: As you inhale, lengthen the body; as you exhale, move opposing arms and legs in small paddling motions for 3-5 breaths, then lower the arms and legs and move into child's pose.

IMPORTANT

Shoulders must be higher than hands! If you are unable to sufficiently extend the spine, simply hold the arms and legs off the floor and skip the paddling motion. Keep the body long and centered! Look at the floor to take stress off the back of the neck.

LEG PULL, FRONT

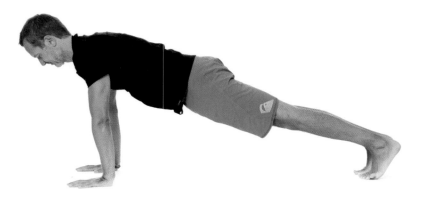

Starting position: Push-up position with legs extended.

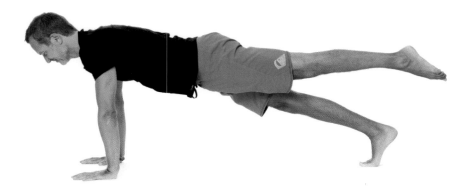

Execution: As you exhale, perform alternating dynamic leg lifts. As you inhale, return the leg to the floor. Repeat 3x per leg.

IMPORTANT

The pelvis is stable. Keep the spine neutral and long. Elbows are soft.

ROLL UP TO STANDING

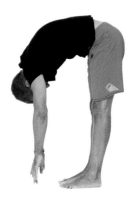

Starting position: Forward bend with feet parallel and hip-width apart.

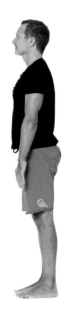

Execution: As you exhale, evenly roll up the spine vertebrae by vertebrae to an upright standing position. Afterwards, perform several shoulder rolls; rest and reflect for several breaths.

IMPORTANT

The abdominal wall remains engaged. Keep the pelvis over the feet. Roll up evenly along the spine and bend the knees if necessary. Let the head hang loosely.

ALL OF THE EXERCISES AT A GLANCE

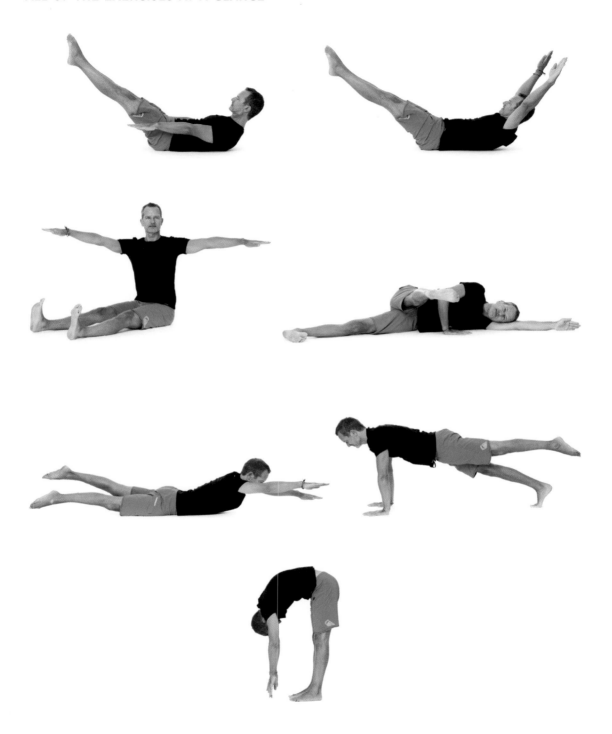

5.3 SILVER MOVER

Human life expectancy is on the rise and that is not likely to change. It is therefore no surprise that the designations for people in the second half of their life are becoming more numerous and more creative: popular coinages are Best Agers, Generation Gold, Golden or Silver Agers. And because this book is about exercise, we have created yet another name, the Silver Mover. Until just a few years ago, people of an advanced age were called Generation 50+. Today this threshold has been moved back quite a bit. According to WHO, people over 65 are considered old. But regardless of how young or old we are, no one can escape the aging process, and it is irreversible. But not everyone ages the same way. While some physically fit seniors mingle at the golf club and can still play 18 holes, some 50-year-olds can barely do a squat. The fact is, we can influence how we age regardless of our genetic disposition. A healthy diet and an appropriate lifestyle with enough sleep and adequate exercise can have a positive effect on our biological age. At age 30, our muscles already begin to lose strength, and at age 50, they start to lose mass. At that time the testosterone level also begins to drop, resulting in additional loss of muscle strength and mass. On the other hand, the percentage of visceral fat increases. The only thing that helps is activity. And it has to start at a young age. People that started to exercise when they were young reduce their risk of muscle loss. According to government statistics, most seniors feel physically fit. And we can start an exercise program accordingly. Needed are multi-joint movements that focus on stability as well as mobility. And even if some people might consider it daring, an intensive strength effort is also necessary to counteract the loss of muscle strength. Most of our muscle loss takes place in the lower extremities. Strength exercises for legs and gluteal muscles are a must, as are mobility exercises for hips and ankles. The upper extremities should maintain their function as the locomotion and support apparatus. The exercises are selected accordingly.

We will introduce Pilates programs for the increasingly larger group of Silver Movers. They differ in terms of intensity and complexity, and are geared to participants with some exercise experience and those interested in exercise or less experienced individuals.

TIPS FOR INSTRUCTORS

The participant's fitness level determines the choice of exercises. A 70-year old active athlete can be much fitter than a 50-year old beginner. Most illnesses in old age affect the cardiovascular system. You should therefore integrate a few minutes of endurance training into your exercise program. Bounce and jump in place, just as Joseph Pilates did years ago.

TIPS FOR STUDENTS

The honeymoon is over! If your physician and trainer have given you a clean bill of health, it's time to get up and get going. Regularity is more important that intensity, which you can gradually increase.

5.3.1   SILVER MOVER: START MOVING PROGRAM

KNEE BOUNCES

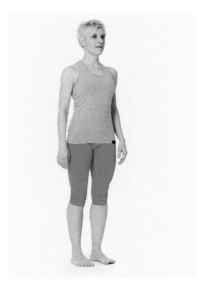

Starting position: Standing position; feet are parallel and hip-width apart.

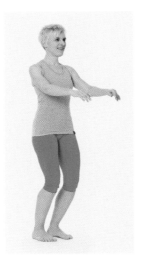
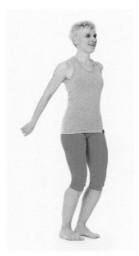

Execution: Loosely bounce in your ankles, knees, and hips; as you do so, rhythmically swing the arms back and forth and take relaxed breaths.

PLEASE NOTE

Bouncing is a strictly vertical movement. The range of motion is small and the upper body remains upright. Watch your hip-knee-foot alignment.

SINGLE-LEG BALANCE

Starting position: Standing position; feet are parallel and hip-width apart.

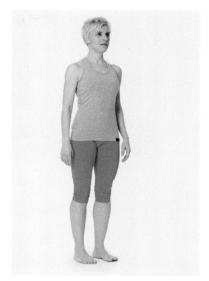

Execution: As you exhale, shift your weight to the right leg and pull the left knee into the body. Hold the left knee with one hand and extend the other arm to the side or use it to hold on to something for support.

As you exhale, externally rotate the left leg from the hip. As you inhale, guide the leg back to the front.

Repeat 6-8x per side.

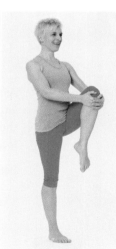
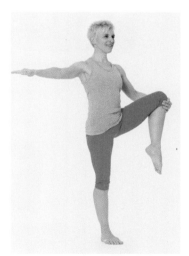

TIP

For a secure stance, fix your eyes on a point in front of you, firmly push the supporting leg into the floor and the crown of the head towards the ceiling to create axial extension.

BASIC BRIDGE WITH KNEE LIFT

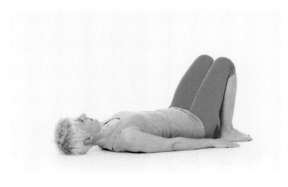

Starting position: On your back with knees bent and feet planted; arms rest alongside the body.

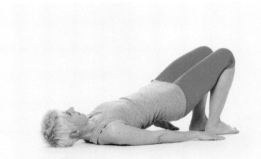

Execution: As you exhale, roll the pelvis up to the shoulder girdle into shoulder bridge.

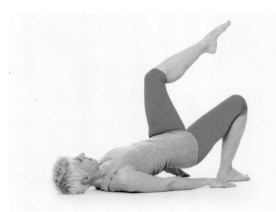

As you exhale, first shift your weight to the right leg. Then lift the left foot off the floor and move the knee towards the body. As you inhale, lower the foot back down to the floor.

Repeat 4x per side.

TIP

In case of cramping in the back of the thigh, it helps to immediately switch sides so the tension continually shifts from side to side. If this works better, the four repetitions per side can be completed back to back.

SCAPULAR REACH

Starting position: On your back with knees bent and feet planted; arms are extended to the ceiling.

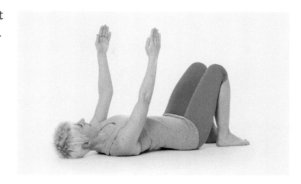

Execution: As you inhale, extend the arms to the ceiling. As you do so, the shoulder blades slide apart and lift off the floor.

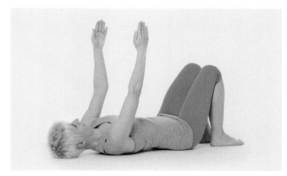

As you exhale, let the shoulder blades drop back down to the floor.

Repeat 4-5x per side.

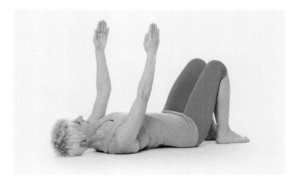

LEG CIRCLE VARIATION: THIGH CIRCLE

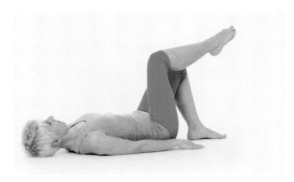

Starting position: On your back; the left foot is planted; the right leg is bent at a 90-degree angle.

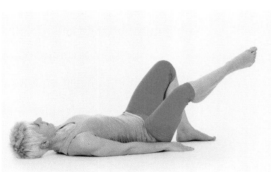

Execution: As you exhale, the right leg circles to the right in a semi-circle and as you inhale, the leg returns to the starting position over the middle of the body.

Repeat 4x per side.

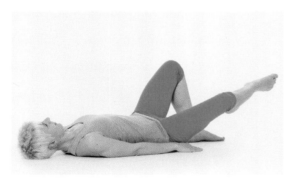

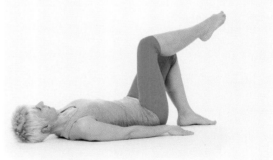

IMPORTANT
The pelvis remains steady.

SIDE KICK

Starting position: On your side; the bottom knee is bent; the top leg is extended and raised to hip level.

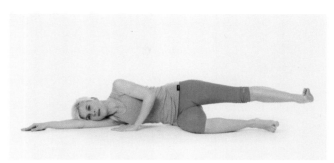

Execution: As you inhale, flex the hip and move the top leg forward. The foot is flexed (dorsal extension).

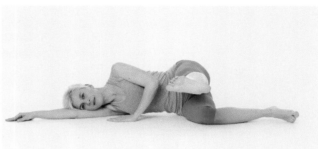

As you exhale, move the leg back in a long arch into hip extension. The foot is pointed.

Repeat 6-8x.

Repeat 4x per side.

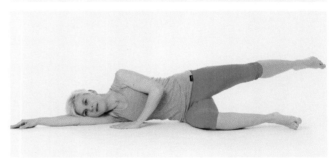

IMPORTANT
The pelvis remains stable. Imagine an air cushion under your waist.

CAT STRETCH

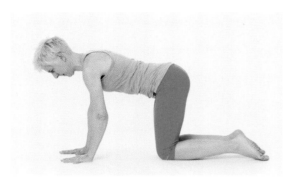

Starting position: On all fours.

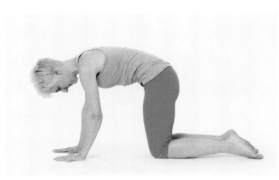

Execution: As you exhale, round the spine from tailbone to the top of the head.

With your next exhalation, extend the spine again, repeat 4-6x, then return to the starting position.

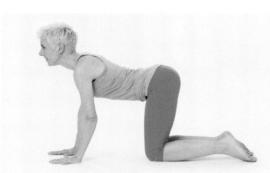

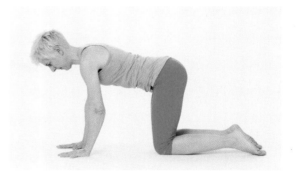

TIP

Rounding the spine is even more pronounced when hands and feet are pressed firmly into the floor. This facilitates a bigger arch. When extending the spine, feet and hands pull towards each other.

ALL OF THE EXERCISES AT A GLANCE

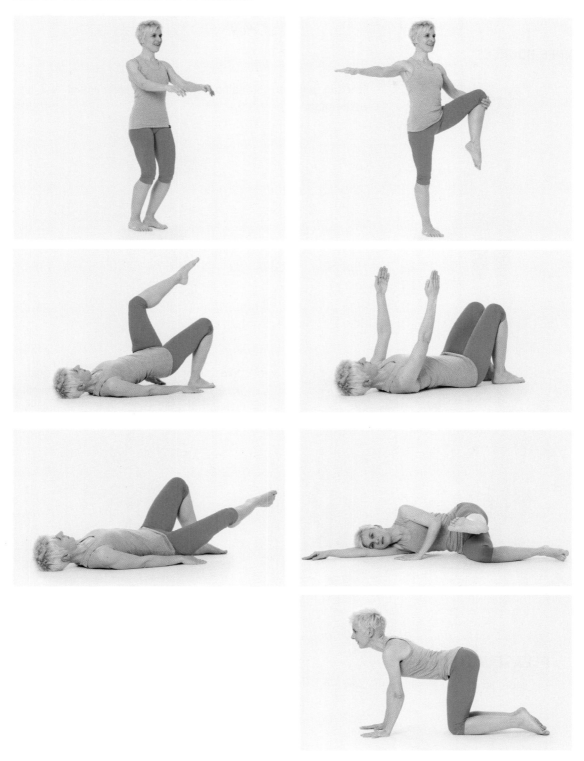

5.3.2 SILVER MOVER: KEEP MOVING PROGRAM

KNEE BOUNCES

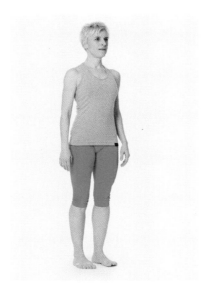

Starting position: Standing position; feet are parallel and hip-width apart.

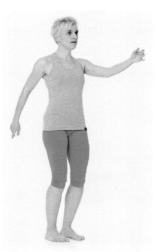
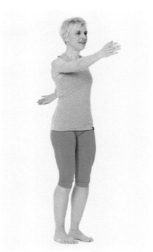

Execution: Loosely bounce in your ankles, knees, and hips; as you do so, rhythmically swing the arms back and forth in opposite directions and take relaxed breaths.

PLEASE NOTE
The shoulder girdle can follow the arm movements and rotate slightly.

SCISSOR JUMPS WITH BOUNCES

Starting position: Standing position, feet are parallel, hip-width apart and in astride position (left foot forward, right foot back).

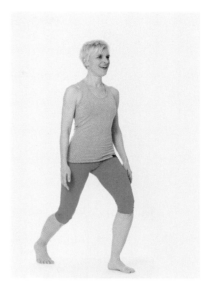

Execution: Bounce 2x with ankles, knees, and hips; arms swing in opposite directions. Then switch leg positions with a jump. Now the right foot is in front. Repeat approximately 10x on opposing diagonals. Take relaxed breaths.

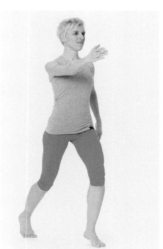
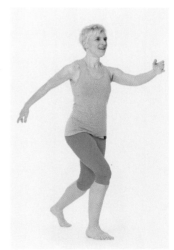

PLEASE NOTE
Arms always move opposite to legs.

BOUNCE TO SINGLE-LEG BALANCE

Starting position: Lunge position with left leg in front.

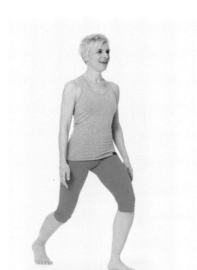

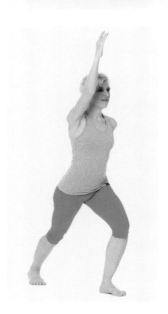 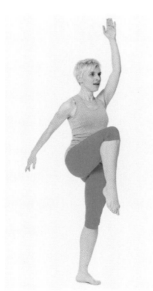

Execution: Push the right heel towards the floor 2x and at the same time alternately extend or pulse the arms to the back, inhaling 2x.

As you exhale, quickly pull the right knee forward and up; arms extend in opposite directions.

Repeat 6-8x per side.

BRIDGING

Starting position: On your back with knees bent and feet planted.

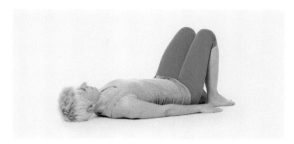

Preparation: As you exhale, roll up into shoulder bridge starting with the tailbone. Then shift your weight to the right leg and extend the left leg to the ceiling.

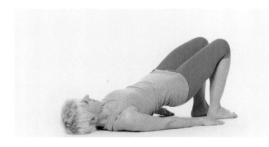

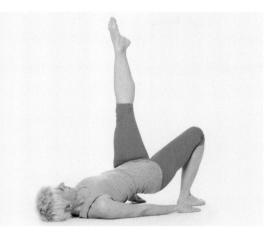

Execution: With the next exhalation, move the extended leg forward in a big arch, as you inhale move it back into a vertical position. Repeat 3-5x per side.

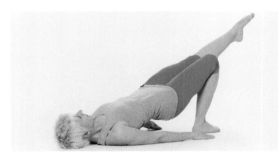

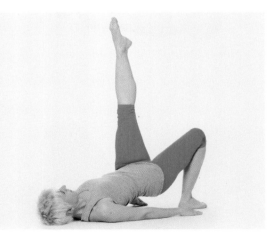

TIP

Actively press the extended arms and the supporting foot into the floor. This creates more stability and body tension.

ARM CIRCLES

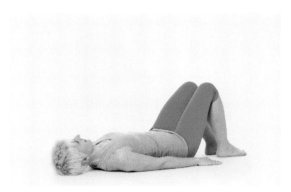

Starting position: On your back with knees bent and feet planted; arms rest alongside the body.

Execution: As you exhale, raise the arms up and overhead in a big arch. As you inhale, laterally lower the arms to the floor and move them back to your sides to the starting position. Repeat 6-8x.

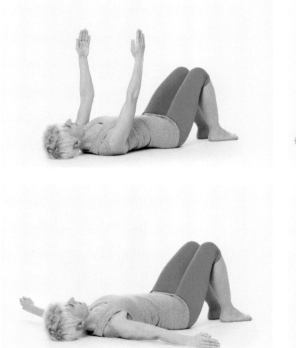

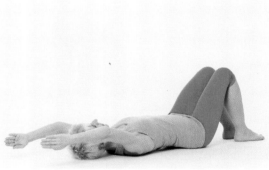

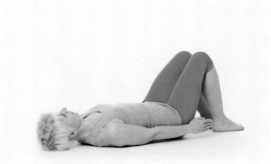

TIP

If you keep your eyes on the ceiling, you will always be able to see your fingertips. This keeps you from making the circle too big, or rather keeps the ribcage from moving.

PLEASE NOTE

The movement takes place only in the shoulder joints. The rear costal arches maintain contact with the floor.

LEG CIRCLE

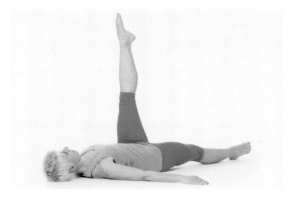

Starting position: On your back, the right leg is extended on the floor; the left leg is extended to the ceiling and slightly externally rotated. The arms rest alongside the body.

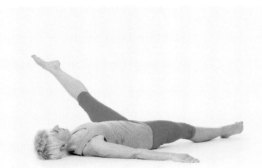

Execution: As you exhale, describe a semi-circle to the outside with the left leg; as you inhale, move the leg back over the midsection.

Repeat 4-6x.

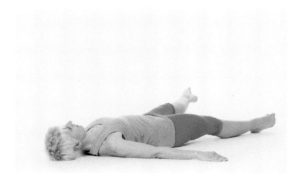

IMPORTANT
The pelvis remains steady.

SIDE KICK

Starting position: On your side, legs are extended at a slight forward angle from the hips.

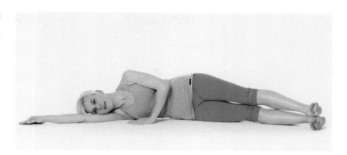

Execution: Flex the hip and move the top leg forward with the foot flexed, and kick 2x at the end of hip flexion. As you do so, take two short breaths.

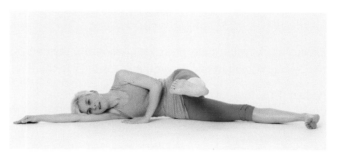

As you exhale, point the foot and move the leg back into hip extension in a long arch.

Repeat 6-8x.

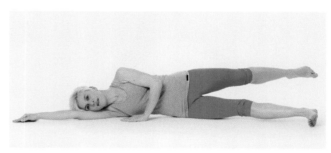

IMPORTANT
The pelvis remains steady. Imagine having an air cushion under your waist.

UP STRETCH

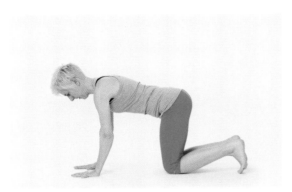

Starting position: On all fours.

Execution: As you exhale, press your hands into the floor, straighten the knees, and lift the pelvis towards the ceiling. As you inhale, lower the knees back to the floor.

Repeat 4-6x.

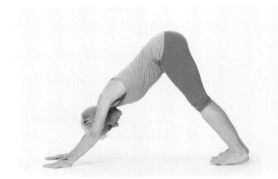 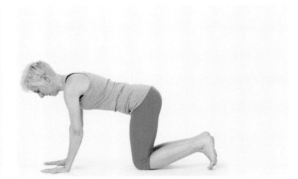

TIP

Imagine your heels pushing into the floor while the sit bones pull up towards the ceiling. This creates length in the back of the legs.

ALL OF THE EXERCISES AT A GLANCE

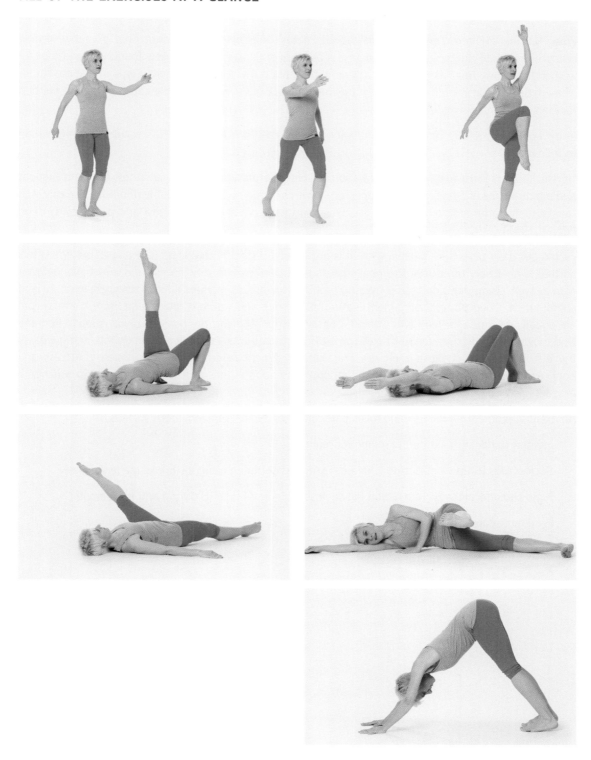

5.4   EXERCISE PROGRAMS FOR MEN

When visiting a Pilates class or hearing about Pilates, one gets the impression that primarily women practice the Pilates method. Reports about the benefits of Pilates are more likely found in magazines for women than men. This has resulted in a general perception that Pilates is a gentle type of gymnastics for women. But Joseph Pilates was actually a gymnast and a boxer who initially created a training method for men.

In his book *Back to Life Through Contrology* published in 1945, Joseph Pilates describes his motivation as follows:

"Physical fitness is the first requisite for happiness. Our interpretation of physical fitness is the attainment and maintenance of a uniformly developed body with a sound mind fully capable of naturally, easily, and satisfactorily performing our many and daily varied tasks with spontaneous zest and pleasure." (Joseph Pilates, 1945)

Facing our daily tasks and mastering them is not a gender-specific challenge. The Pilates method offers all that is necessary to achieve this goal. The mat exercises can be very intense and are challenging for men as well. Using one's body as a training tool in the exercises requires a lot of strength, mobility, and coordination. Good physical alignment, natural breathing, and vigorous movements from a strong core are equally desirable for men and women. Consciously lengthening the body (two-way stretch, Romana Kryzanowska) during the exercises takes stress off joints, improves range of motion (ROM), and increases the effectiveness of strength exercises. Practicing in functional units increases exercise success and application in everyday life. Mobility and strength are adapted, increased, and improved in functional amounts according to the student's needs.

An exercise program for men should focus particularly on typical problem areas such as:

- Lumbar spine (stiffness during rolling movements)
- Back of legs (tight when sitting with legs extended or during exercises like single-leg circles)
- Rigid shoulders (kinetic interaction between scapula and humerus during arm movements)
- Current discomforts
- Old injuries
- Excess weight

Men have a tendency to work out too hard and overexert the body. "No pain, no gain" and "more is better" are common thought patterns. Idealized body images of washboard abs and broad shoulders might be a good motivator to start exercising, but when they lead to over-exercising they get in the way of success.

A lack of body sense must be taken into account when teaching the exercises, but flowery language should be avoided.

For overweight participants, the trunk must be prepared via Pilates pre-exercises to avoid overloading of the low back.

Men generally have stronger arms and shoulders, so more supporting exercises can be incorporated.

TIPS FOR INSTRUCTORS

Take into account any existing restrictions of range of motion, particularly in the hips and spine. If necessary, find alternative starting positions (e.g., for sitting with legs extended) or use aids (cushions, towels, etc.). You can incorporate light hand weights (up to 2 kg (4.4 lbs.)) for advanced participants. Forgo flowery descriptions and dance-like movements.

TIPS FOR STUDENTS

Focus on the best-possible execution and accept aids. Push to your limit, but not beyond. More is not always better, and the old saying that you cannot succeed without pain is not good advice. Complete the exercises you'd rather skip, with joy and concentration.

5.4.1   PROGRAM 1 FOR MEN

CAT STRETCH

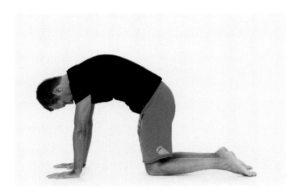

Starting position: On all fours with hands below shoulders and knees below hips.

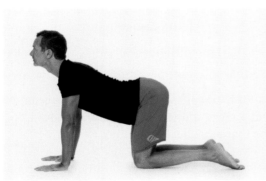

Execution: As you exhale, round the back from the tailbone to the top of the head and as you inhale, return to the starting position or a gently arched back. Repeat 5-6x.

Variation: After three repetitions, reverse the breathing pattern.

TIP

Look towards your cheekbones when you round the back and towards your eyebrows when you extend or arch the back!

IMPORTANT

Move the spine evenly. Elbows are soft. Abdominal muscles are engaged.

ONE HUNDRED

Starting position: On your back with closed, raised legs; knees are bent approximately 90 degrees above the hips; hands are next to the body.

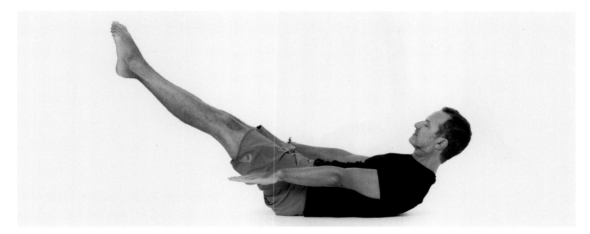

Execution: As you exhale, reach towards your feet with your hands; upon exhalation, roll up head and shoulders to the shoulder girdle while simultaneously extending the legs. As you exhale again, begin to vigorously pump the arms up and down. Pump 5x per inhalation and exhalation. Repeat up to 10x.

TIP
Look towards your thighs and pelvis.

IMPORTANT
Trunk and shoulders remain stable. Depending on your level of mobility and abdominal strength, extend the legs and move them closer to the floor.

SUPINE LEG STRETCH

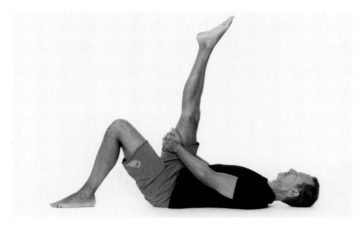

Starting position: On your back with one leg propped on the floor and the other leg extended to the ceiling; hands grip the thigh.

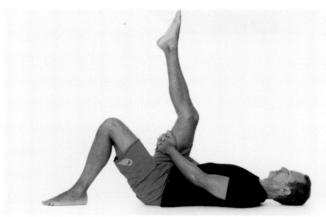

Execution: As you exhale, straighten the leg and as you inhale, slightly bend the knee again. Repeat 3x, each time deepening the stretch. Then switch legs.

Variation: Extend the supporting leg on the floor.

TIP
Use a towel or something similar to lengthen the arms.

IMPORTANT
Maintain a neutral supine position. Shoulder blades remain on the floor.

SINGLE-LEG STRETCH

Starting position: On your back; the upper body is rolled up to the shoulder blades (sternum drop); both legs are bent and raised off the floor, hands grip the lower legs.

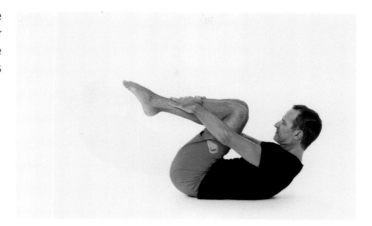

Execution: As you exhale, extend the left leg forward and hold on to the right leg with both hands. As you inhale, start to extend the right leg and bend the left leg. As you exhale again, extend the right leg and hold on to the lower left leg with both hands. Repeat 3-5x per leg.

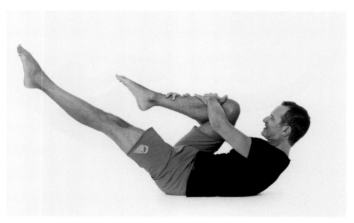

TIP
Move your legs in parallel as though they are on tracks.

IMPORTANT
The upper body remains stable. Extend the legs at approximately a 45-degree angle. Move rhythmically and evenly.

CRISS-CROSS

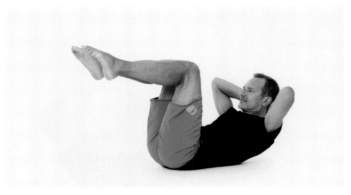

Starting position: On your back, the upper body is rolled up to the shoulder blades; both legs are bent and raised off the floor; hands are folded at the back of the head.

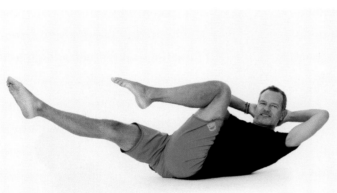

Execution: As you exhale, extend the left leg forward and roll the right elbow back. As you inhale, return to the starting position. With the next exhalation, initiate the motion sequence on the other side. Repeat 3-5x per leg.

TIP

Turn your head and gaze towards the elbow that rolls back. Focus on the extension part of the movement and not the convergence of the elbow and knee.

SPINAL STRETCH

Starting position: Sit with your legs extended forward and slightly more than shoulder-width apart; arms are extended forward parallel at shoulder-level.

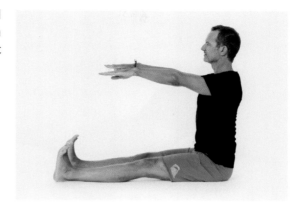

Execution: As you exhale, roll forward vertebrae by vertebrae starting with the head. The arms remain parallel to the floor and the head stays above the arms. As you inhale, roll back up to an upright position. Repeat 3x.

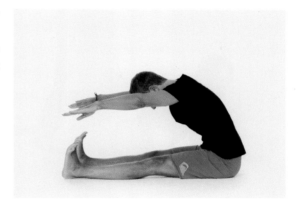

TIP

Imagine you are sitting against a wall—or actually sit against a wall. Peel off the wall to roll forward, and then roll back up against the wall. Look in the direction of movement.

SINGLE-LEG KICK

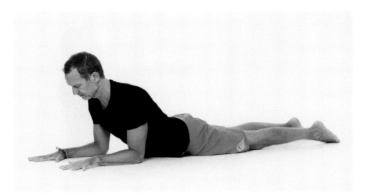

Starting position: Cobra resting on the forearms.

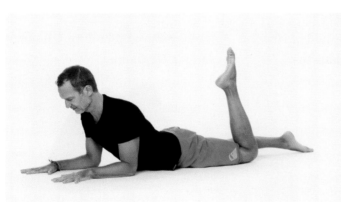

Execution: As you exhale, activate the core, lift the sternum, and firmly press the forearms into the floor. As you inhale, kick the left heel 2x towards the left sit bone (two quick breaths); as you exhale, extend the leg and lower it back to the floor. Repeat the sequence with the right leg. Repeat 3-5x per leg.

IMPORTANT

The pelvis remains on the floor and the hip is extended. Vigorously press the arms into the floor and organize the shoulder girdle. Stay centered and keep the body long. Extend the leg from the hip far enough so the kneecap doesn't rub against the floor. Keep an eye on leg alignment.

SWIMMING

Starting position: On your stomach with arms extended forward on either side of the head and legs extended back.

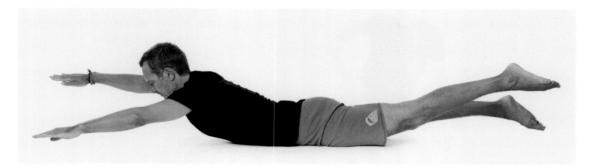

Execution: As you exhale, lift first the upper body, then both arms and legs off the floor. As you inhale, lengthen the body, then exhale and simultaneously paddle arms and legs with short strokes on a diagonal. Keep moving for 3-5 breaths, then return to the floor and move into child's pose.

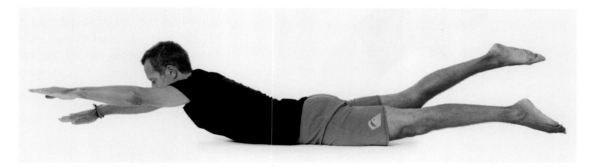

IMPORTANT

Shoulders must be higher than the hands! If your extension is not adequate yet, simply hold everything off the floor and skip the paddling motion. Stay long and centered! Look at the floor to take pressure off the back of the neck!

SIDE BEND

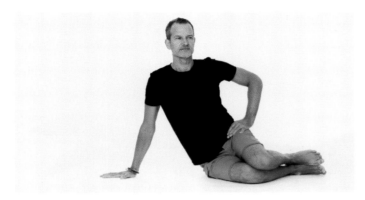

Starting position: Sit sideways on the right hip with knees bent; the right hand is propped next to you on the floor with fingers pointing away from the body; the left hand rests against the left hip.

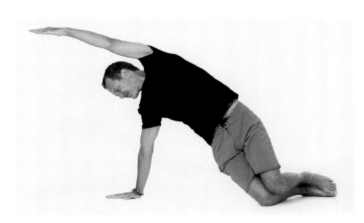

Execution: As you exhale, firmly press the right hand into the floor, activate the core, and move your body into a long arch from the knees to the top of the head. As you do so, extend the left arm overhead. Look at your right hand. As you inhale, move back into the starting position with a controlled motion. Repeat 2x, then switch sides.

IMPORTANT

Imagine sitting against a wall. Vigorously push off the floor with hands and feet during the entire movement; stay centered and keep the body long; keep the shoulder blades integrated and the elbows gently extended.

PUSH-UP

Starting position: Push-up position with legs extended.

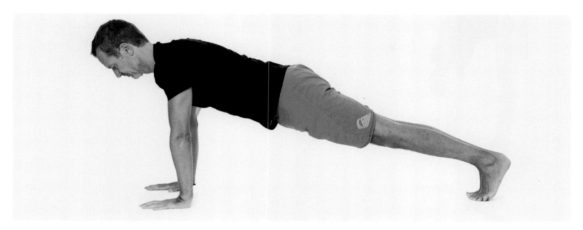

Execution: As you exhale, bend the elbows approximately 90 degrees and straighten them again as you inhale. Repeat 3-8x.

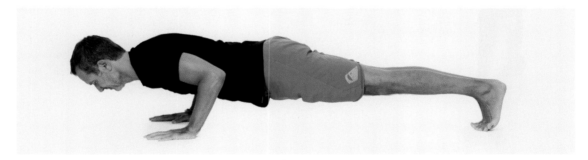

IMPORTANT

Keep the pelvis steady and the spine neutral; keep the body centered and long; bend the elbows close to the body towards the pelvis; when the arms are extended, the shoulder blades lie against the ribcage.

ROLL UP TO STANDING AND SHOULDER ROLLS

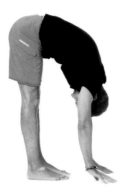

Starting position: Forward bend.

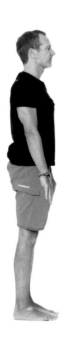

Execution: As you exhale, roll up vertebrae by vertebrae to an upright standing position.

Afterwards, do a few shoulder rolls, then rest and reflect for several breaths.

IMPORTANT

Keep the abdominal wall activated. Keep the pelvis over the feet. Roll evenly along the spine and if necessary bend the knees. Allow the head to hang loosely.

ALL OF THE EXERCISES AT A GLANCE

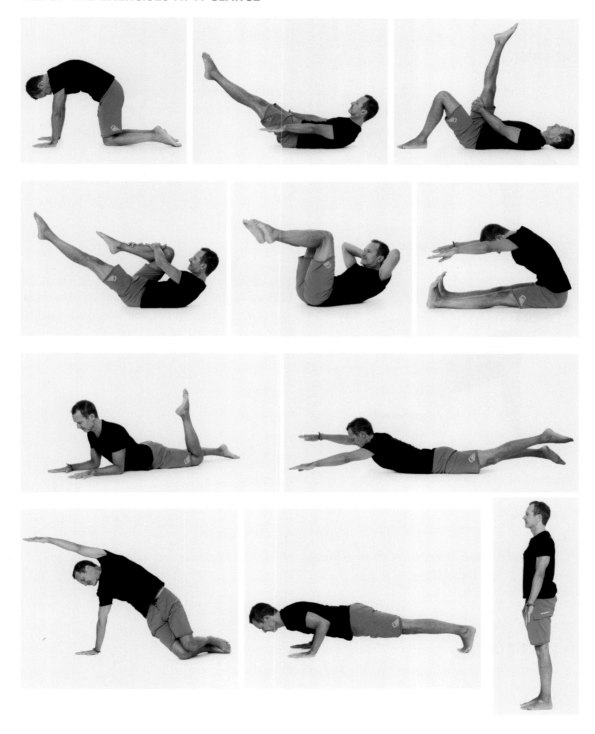

5.4.2   PROGRAM 2 FOR MEN

CAT STRETCH

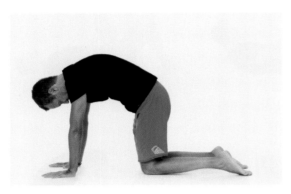

Starting position: On all fours with hands below shoulders and knees below hips.

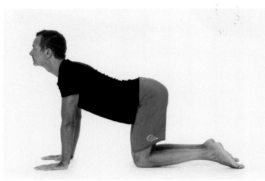

Execution: As you exhale, round the back from the tailbone to the top of the head and as you inhale, return to the starting position or a gently arched back. Repeat 5-6x.

Variation: After three repetitions, reverse the breathing pattern.

TIP
Look towards your cheekbones when you round the back and towards your eyebrows when you extend or arch the back!

IMPORTANT
Move the spine evenly. Elbows are soft. Abdominal muscles are engaged.

ROLL UP

Starting position: On your back with legs extended; arms rest alongside the body.

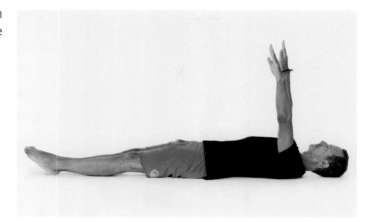

Execution: As you inhale, lift the arms so they are stacked over the shoulders; as you exhale, roll up vertebrae by vertebrae starting with the head all the way to the sit bones until the upper body is extended over the legs in a long even arch.

With your next inhalation, roll back down vertebrae by vertebrae. Repeat 3-4x.

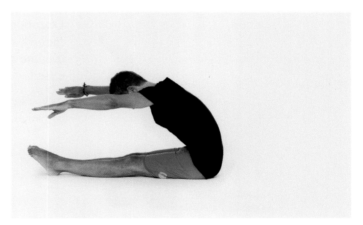

TIP

Look in the direction of movement; if necessary, cushion the spine.

ROLL OVER

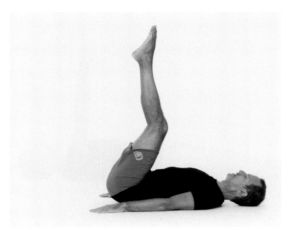

Starting position: On your back with feet planted on the floor and arms extended alongside the body.

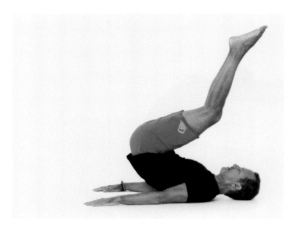

Execution: As you exhale, move the knees towards the body one at a time until the knees are positioned over the hips. Knees are slightly bent and legs are closed.

As you exhale, roll the pelvis up off the floor, and as you inhale, roll it back down. Repeat 3x.

IMPORTANT

Do not use leg momentum. The back of the neck stays long. Shoulder blades remain on the floor. Fingertips reach towards the front edge of the mat.

DOUBLE-LEG STRETCH

Starting position: On your back; roll the upper body up to the shoulder blades (sternum drop); both knees are bent in the air and hands rest on the shins.

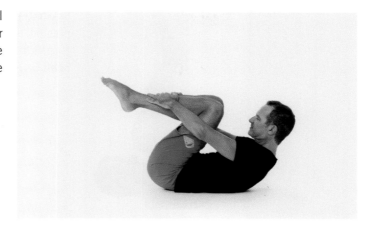

Execution: As you exhale, extend the closed legs forward at a 45-degree angle and extend the arms parallel towards the head at the same angle. As you inhale, circle the arms to the outside; when the arms are at approximately shoulder level, bend the knees and return to the starting position. Repeat 3-5x.

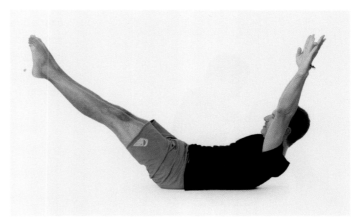

IMPORTANT
The upper body remains steady. Move rhythmically and evenly.

ROLLING BACK

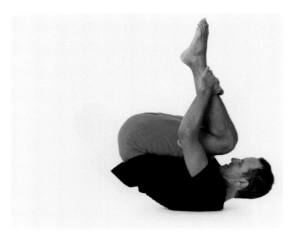

Starting position: Sit with your knees bent and feet planted; hands grip the shins; the upper body forms a perfect arch from the tailbone to the top of the head.

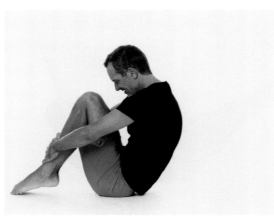

Execution: As you exhale, pull the heels close to your bottom and balance on your sacrum. As you inhale, roll back to the shoulder girdle. As you exhale, roll back up into your balancing pose. Repeat 6-8x.

IMPORTANT

Actively pull the abdominal wall away from the thighs. Maintain the ball shape throughout the entire motion sequence. Do not use momentum from the legs, and don't roll onto the head.

SAW

Starting position: Sit with legs extended and slightly more than mat-width apart; arms are laterally extended at shoulder level, palms face the floor.

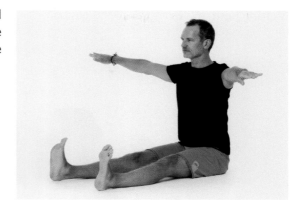

Execution: As you inhale, lengthen the spine and rotate the upper body to the left. The right arm externally rotates and the left arm internally rotates. As you exhale, roll your upper body forward vertebrae by vertebrae, and as you do so, reach with your right pinkie towards the left little toe. As you inhale, roll back to your seated position and continue to rotate left. As you exhale, return to the starting position. Repeat 3x per side.

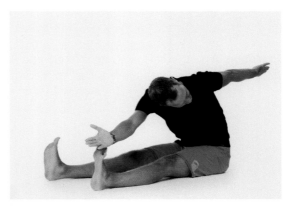

IMPORTANT

Sit evenly on both sit bones during the entire movement sequence and keep them firmly anchored to the mat. Don't let the upper body drop onto the legs but keep it actively suspended. This is primarily a stretch for the spine and not the legs.

SIDE-LYING DOUBLE-LEG LIFT, ABDUCTION AND ADDUCTION

Starting position: Neutral side-lying position.

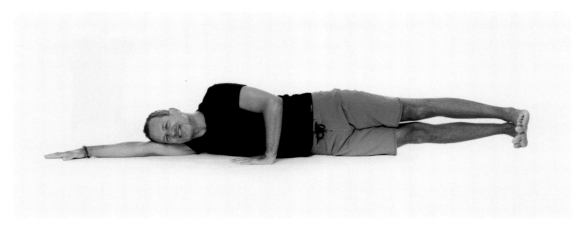

Execution: As you exhale, activate the core and the adductors and slightly raise the closed legs off the floor. As you inhale, lower the legs back to the starting position. Repeat 5-8x.

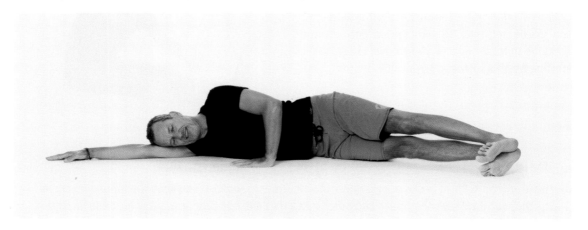

Then move the closed legs slightly forward of the pelvis and lower them to the mat.

As you exhale, vigorously lift the top leg up off the bottom leg and as you inhale, push it back down against an imaginary resistance. Repeat 3-5x.

Switch sides.

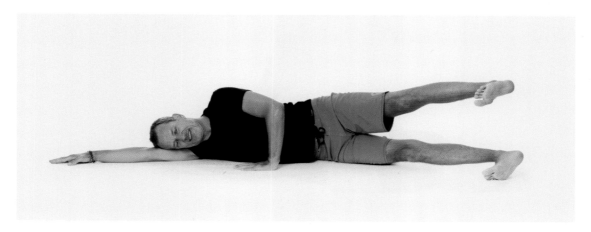

IMPORTANT

The weight of the trunk is distributed between the pelvis and the ribcage, not the area in between. Use a pillow if you lack the shoulder mobility to rest your head on the extended arm. Place a rolled-up towel under the waist for more length. Keep the body long and centered!

DOUBLE-LEG KICK

Starting position: On your stomach with legs extended and closed; hands rest on top of each other in the hollow of the low back; elbows are bent and hang down at your sides; the head rests on one side.

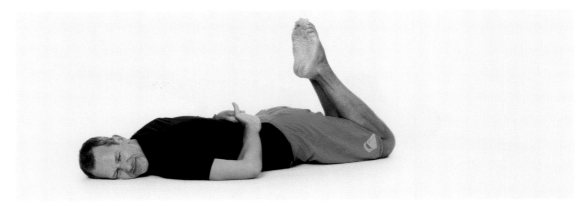

Execution: As you inhale, kick your heels 2-3x towards your bottom; as you exhale, vigorously extend both legs and simultaneously extend the arms towards the feet and lift the upper body while turning the head towards the mat; as you inhale, turn the head to the other side and rest it on the mat; at the same time bend the elbows and return to the starting position. Still inhaling, vigorously kick the heels towards your bottom again. Repeat 3x per side.

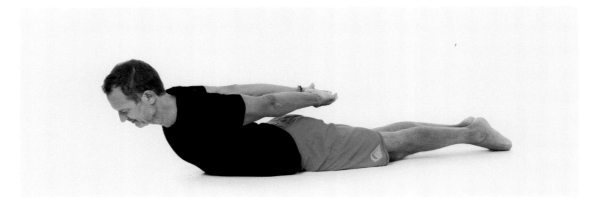

TIP
Lower the upper body back down to the mat before kicking again. Imagine the hands, feet, and head being connected for a fluid extending and lifting movement.

SWAN DIVE

Starting position: On your stomach, legs are extended and hands are planted next to the ribcage.

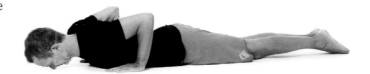

Execution: As you exhale, lift the upper body off the floor in a long arch. Lengthen the body as you inhale and create a strong line from the soles of the feet to the back of the head. As you exhale, start to lower the upper body while simultaneously lifting the legs off the floor. Inhale and reverse the sequence. Repeat 3-5x, then move into child's pose.

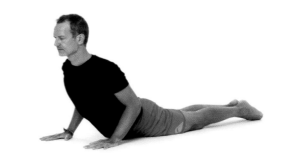

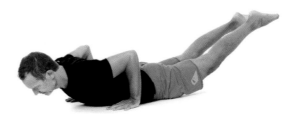

TIP

Imitate the movements of a rocking horse. This movement is not particularly accommodating of a man's anatomy. Adjust yourself before rocking.

SINGLE-LEG TEASER

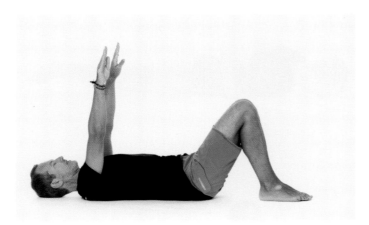

Starting position: On your back, arms are extended alongside the body, palms down, and the feet are planted in extension of the sit bones.

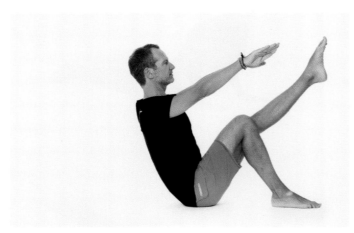

Execution: As you inhale, raise the arms towards the ceiling. With the next exhalation, activate your abdominal muscles and roll up vertebrae by vertebrae to the base of the spine. Simultaneously extend your left leg (keep the knees closed) and extend the arms forward parallel to the left leg. With your next exhalation, return to the starting position. Repeat with the right leg. Repeat 3x per leg.

IMPORTANT

Keep the shoulders wide and the back of the neck long. Lead with the sternum as you come up, but keep the lumbar spine rounded. Create length with the top of the head, heel, and fingertips. Keep the inner-thigh muscles engaged and firmly anchor the supporting foot on the floor. The abdominal muscles stay engaged throughout the movement.

LEG PULL, FRONT

Starting position: Push-up position with legs extended.

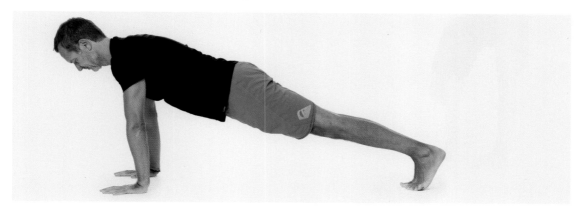

Execution: As you exhale, lift one leg off the floor in a dynamic motion and lower it back down as you inhale, alternating legs. Repeat 3x per leg.

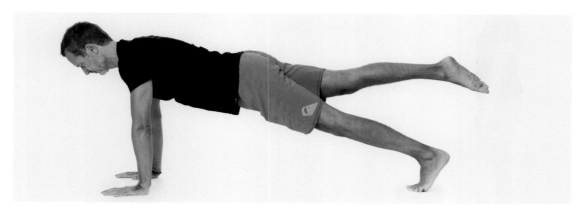

IMPORTANT
Keep the pelvis steady, the spine neutral and long, and the elbows soft.

ROLL UP TO STANDING AND SHOULDER ROLLS

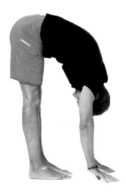

Starting position: Forward bend.

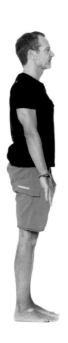

Execution: As you exhale, straighten the legs and roll up vertebrae by vertebrae into an upright standing position.

Afterwards, do several shoulder rolls, then rest and reflect for several breaths.

IMPORTANT

The abdominal wall stays activated (no leg stretches!). Keep the pelvis over the feet. Roll evenly along the spine and if necessary bend the knees. Allow the head to hang loosely.

ALL OF THE EXERCISES AT A GLANCE

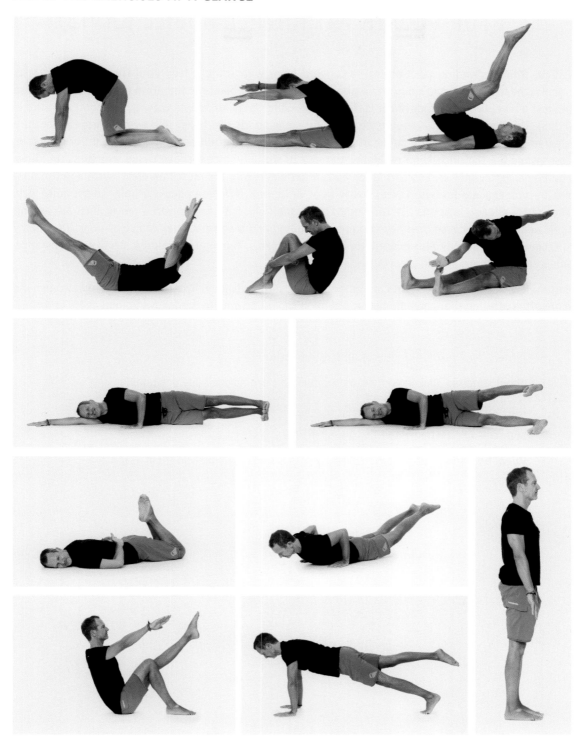

5.5 CLEOPATRA (EXERCISE SEQUENCE FOR PEOPLE WITH HYPERMOBILE JOINTS)

Rolling from a standing position into a forward bend with straight legs until the upper body rests against the legs, doing the splits as a warm-up, being able to bend the fingers in every direction. These are just a few examples of movements that are like child's play for people with hypermobility syndrome (HMS). This phenomenon is even a necessity for some sports like ballet and gymnastics, to meet the ideal image. Even among the public at large, hypermobility is often perceived as elegant or desirable. Less visible are the underlying problems: the lack of stability in connective tissue structures (tendons, ligaments, joint capsules, and cartilage) leads to problems with the musculoskeletal system. Additional health problems are bruises, a weak pelvic floor, or hernias. Affected people usually adjust quite well. They rarely engage in sports like running or track and field. Fast and powerful movements are among their weak spots because they have trouble controlling and stabilizing their joint positions. They enjoy stretching but that may also exacerbate existing problems. Terminal, long stretches like, for instance, some yoga positions should be avoided.

Fortunately, most of our class participants tend to only have individual hypermobile joints, and women are more often affected than men. Particular attention should be paid to the following joints:

- Elbows (hyperextension during supporting positions)

- Shoulder joints (lack of control in overhead and behind-the-body positions)

- Knees (bow legs, knock knees)

- Lumbar spine (extreme arch)

- Wrists and fingers (pain during supporting positions or cannot do them at all)

Hypermobile participants need lots of help in finding the correct joint position. The joints have so-called blind spots, meaning the affected individuals have little body awareness in the correct joint position and struggle to control and stabilize them. Stabilizing exercises with light weights are helpful, whereby the starting position, particularly for supporting exercises, needs to be modified.

TIPS FOR INSTRUCTORS

Avoid terminal movements, offer additional exercises for body awareness and also use light weights or wrist and ankle weights. Absolutely enforce the correct starting position and exercise execution.

TIPS FOR STUDENTS

Accept the challenge and focus on the exercises you have probably avoided so far. While being flexible certainly feels good, in the long term it is only sustainable with the right amount of physical stability.

THE PROGRAM FOR PEOPLE WITH HYPERMOBILE JOINTS

LOW ABS I

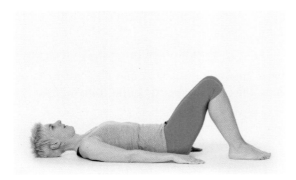

Starting position: On your back with knees bent and feet planted.

Execution: As you exhale, move the left knee towards the body until hip and knee form a 90-degree angle. With your next exhalation, return to the starting position.

Repeat 4-5x, alternating sides.

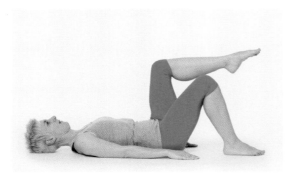 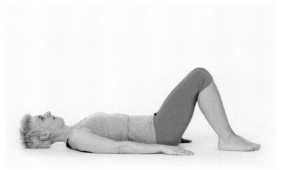

IMPORTANT
Hold the pelvis steady on the floor.

STERNUM DROP

Starting position: On your back with knees bent and feet planted.

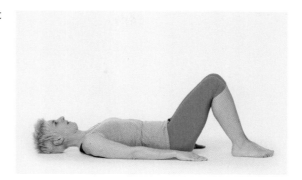

Execution: As you exhale, reach with your hands towards your feet, then roll head and shoulders up to the shoulder girdle. As you inhale, roll back down to the starting position.

Repeat 6-8x.

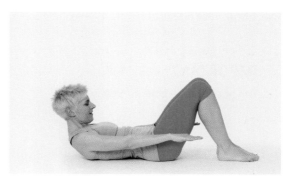

IMPORTANT

Keep the pelvis in its neutral position. The sit bones point towards the heels.

ONE HUNDRED I

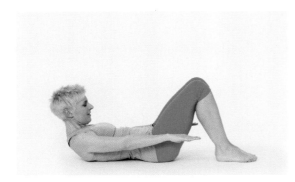

Starting position: On your back with knees bent and feet planted; the upper body is rolled up (sternum drop); arms are extended alongside the body.

Execution: Take 5 short breaths, then exhale 5x in short bursts. Fan the arms in time with the breath.

IMPORTANT
The upper body remains steady.

LOW ABS II

Starting position: On your back with knees bent and feet planted.

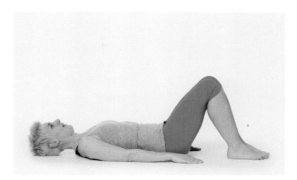

Execution: As you exhale, move the knees towards the body one at a time until knees and hips form a 90-degree angle. With the next exhalation, lower the feet back down to the floor one at a time.

Repeat 4-5x, alternating sides.

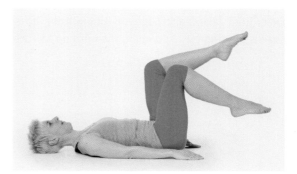

IMPORTANT
The pelvis remains steady on the floor, particularly while lifting the second leg.

ONE HUNDRED II

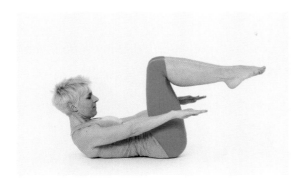

Starting position: On your back, legs are in a 90/90-degree position; the upper body is rolled up (sternum drop); arms are extended alongside the body.

Execution: Take 5 short breaths through the nose and exhale 5x in short bursts through the mouth or nose while vigorously pumping the arms up to 100x; then roll head, arms, and legs back down to the mat.

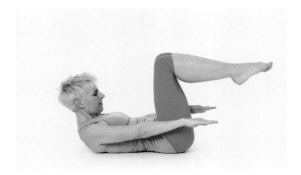 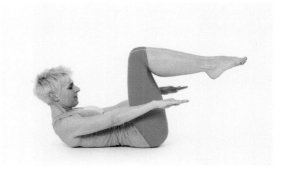

IMPORTANT
The upper body remains steady.

BRIDGE

Starting position: Shoulder bridge.

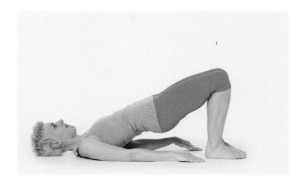

Execution: As you exhale, shift your weight to the right leg and move the left knee towards the body. As you inhale, return to the starting position.

Repeat 6-8x, alternating sides.

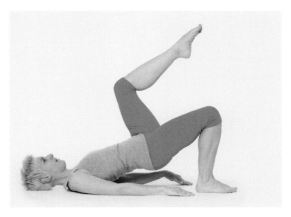

ROLL UP

Starting position: On your back; one leg is extended, the other knee is bent, and the foot is planted.

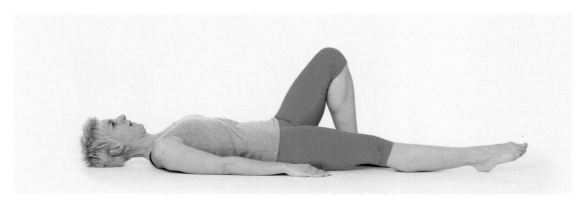

Execution: As you exhale, roll up starting with the head until the shoulder girdle is positioned over the pelvic girdle.

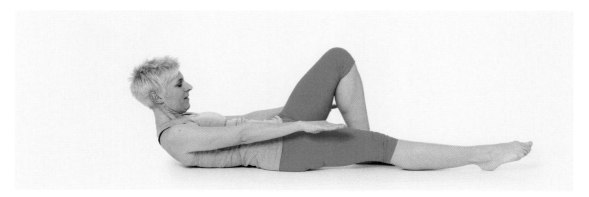

Then lift the spine. With the next exhalation, roll back down to the starting position beginning with the pelvis.

Repeat 4-6x.

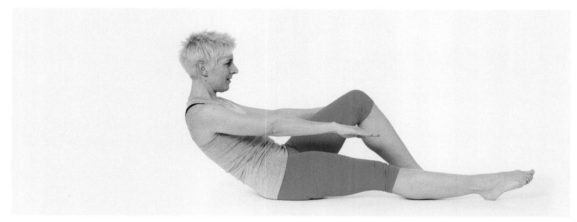

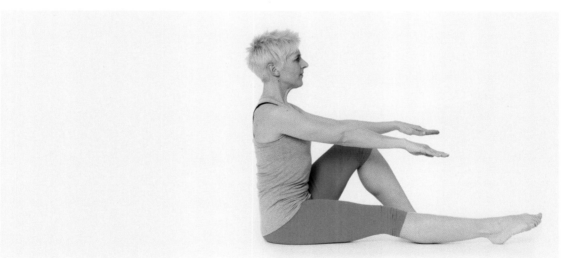

PLEASE NOTE

The motion sequence should be fluid and even.

SWIMMER

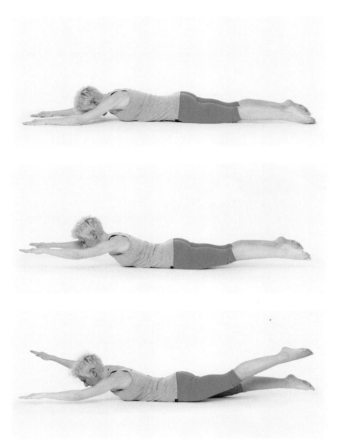

Starting position: On your stomach, arms are extended forward. Arms and legs are slightly raised.

Execution: Briskly paddle arms and legs on a diagonal. Continue to breathe evenly.

KNEE LIFT

Starting position: On all fours.

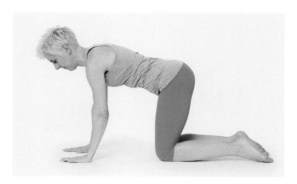

Execution: As you exhale, the abdominal wall first pulls in towards the low back (centering) and the hands press into the floor. Next lift the knees off the floor. As you inhale, lower the knees back down to the floor.

Repeat 6-8x.

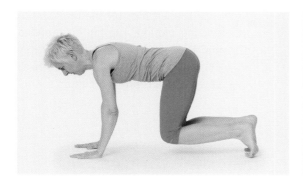
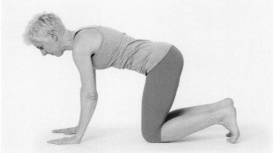

IMPORTANT
Stay centered and maintain muscle tension in the shoulder girdle. Do not hyperextend the elbows.

LEG PULL, FRONT VARIATION

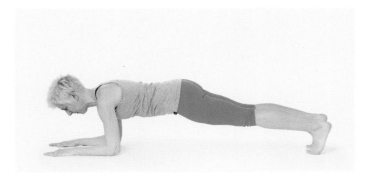

Starting position: Forearm plank.

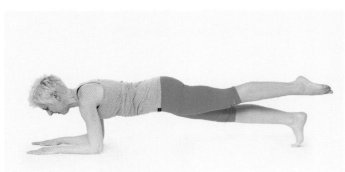

Execution: With each exhalation, press the forearms into the floor so the shoulder girdle is activated. Then shift your weight to the right leg and raise the left foot off the floor with a swiping motion. The hip is extended and the leg springs back and slightly up. As you inhale, lower the leg back down with a controlled motion.

Repeat 4-6x, alternating legs.

IMPORTANT

The pelvis remains steady. Stay centered and keep the spine long.

SWIMMER VARIATION KNEELING

Starting position: On your knees, arms are extended forward. Lean back with a straight back and hips extended (hinge back). You should feel a definite pull in the front of the thighs.

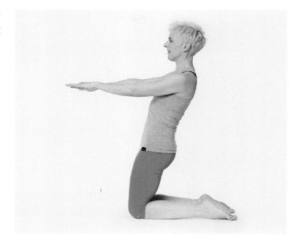

Execution: Paddle the arms up and down with short opposing strokes. As you do so, open the arms to the sides and bring them back together with even arm movements. Keep breathing evenly.

Repeat 4-5x.

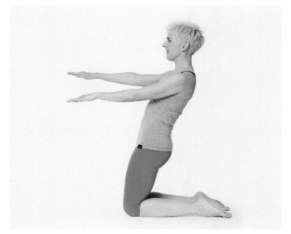

IMPORTANT
Maintain the kneeling position (hinge back).

STANDING LEG BALANCE

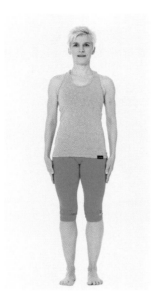

Starting position: Standing.

Execution: As you exhale, shift your weight to your right leg and move the left knee towards the body. Grip the knee and flex the hip as much as possible without shifting the pelvis. The left sit bone actively pulls down. Next, guide the leg to the outside in external rotation with each exhalation, and then across the center of the body in internal rotation. Repeat with the left leg.

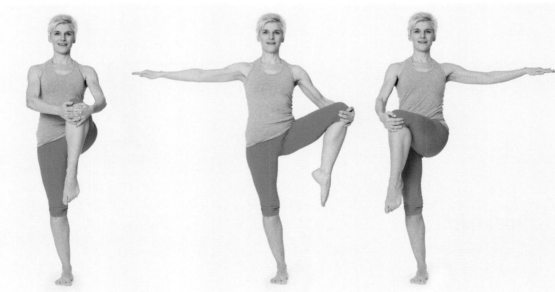

IMPORTANT

The supporting leg and hip remain steady.

ALL OF THE EXERCISES AT A GLANCE

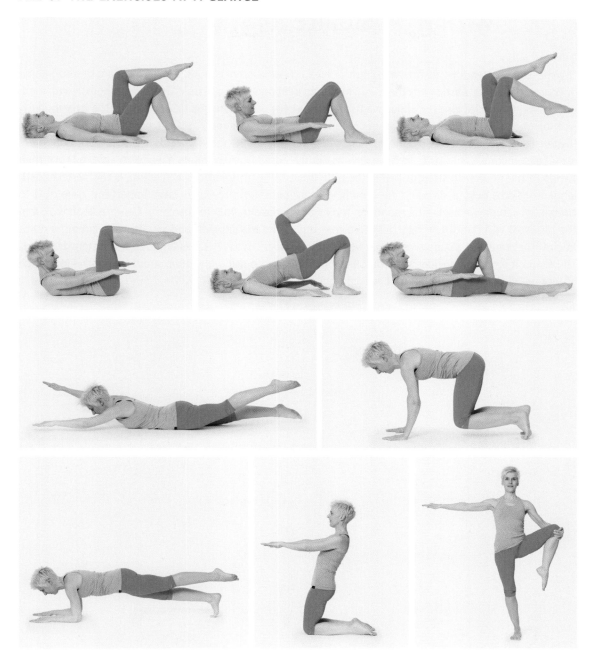

5.6 VIKINGS (EXERCISE SEQUENCE FOR PEOPLE WITH HYPOMOBILE JOINTS)

"My muscles and tendons are extremely tight," "I really need to stretch more." Have you heard this from some of your participants, particularly men? You might be dealing with a classic Viking type. A person with more and stronger muscles whose connective tissue is rigid and subcutaneous tissue is tight. The hypomobility phenomenon (hypo: under/below) is quite normal and just as common as the hypermobility phenomenon (hyper: excessive). But it mostly affects men, whereas women tend more towards hypermobility. But before we label someone as too stiff, we have to consider the norm. Does everyone have to be able to touch their hands to the floor with straight legs or be able to sit tall with their legs extended? Is the perfect cross-legged or Lotus pose a standard for a body with average flexibility? It is more important to be able to complete everyday movements: squatting, looking over the shoulder in the car or being able to look into the backseat without discomfort, getting dishes out of the top cabinet, and smoothly absorbing a quick hop off the stepstool. Viking types more frequently experience torn Achilles tendons and frozen shoulders. The exercise program includes stretches. Slow, melting, and pulsing, dynamic stretches use the full range of motion all the way to the limit of stretching ability.

TIP FOR INSTRUCTORS

Encourage your participants to do more feminine-appearing movements and body-awareness exercises.

TIP FOR STUDENTS

"Little strokes fell big oaks." Only regular practice will help you become more flexible.

THE PROGRAM FOR PEOPLE WITH HYPOMOBILE JOINTS

STRETCHNG THE FRONTAL LINE

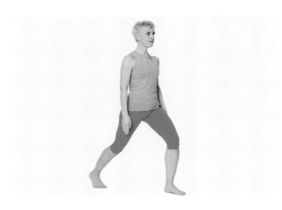

Starting position: Step into a high lunge; left leg in front; left knee is bent; right leg is extended back.

Execution: As you inhale, move the arms forward and overhead, and extend the spine. The gaze is directed diagonally upward, creating a stretch in the entire right front.

As you exhale, round the spine into a big arch, bend the knees, and extend the arms back in a counter pose. Repeat 6-8x per side.

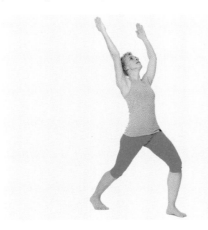
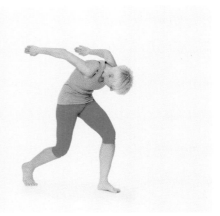

IMPORTANT
Avoid hyperextending the lumbar spine (arched back). Stay centered even as you inhale.

TIP
Add little pulses at the end of extension to deepen the stretch.

SIDE BEND STANDING

Starting position: Standing; the left leg is crossed over the right leg; arms are extended to the ceiling.

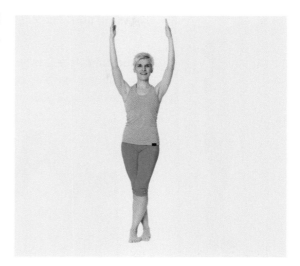

Execution: As you exhale, shift the pelvis to the right. The arms reach into space. The body forms an elongated crescent shape, stretching the entire right side of the body. As you inhale, return to the starting position.

Repeat 6-8x per side.

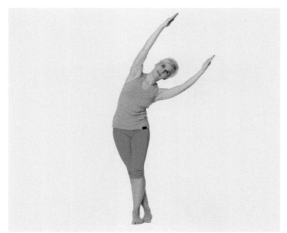

TIP
Add little pulses at the end of the stretch to deepen the stretch.

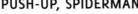 **PILATES**

PUSH-UP, SPIDERMAN

Starting position: Standing.

Execution: As you exhale, roll the spine down; as you inhale, walk your hands forward into push-up position. As you exhale, lift the hips into up stretch; as you inhale, walk your hands to your feet; exhale and roll back up to standing.

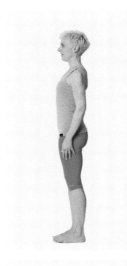
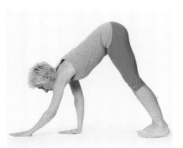
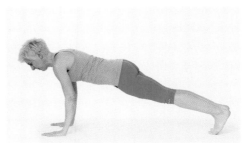

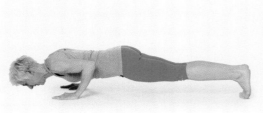
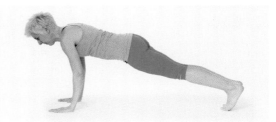

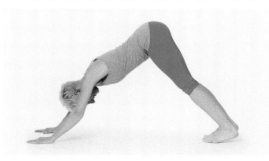

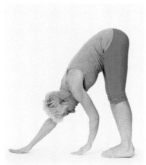
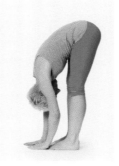
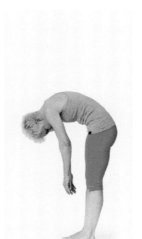
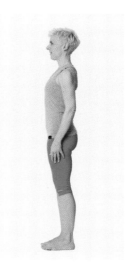

Variation 1: From up stretch, move the left foot to the outside of the left hand with one big step. The right hip is now extended. Now push the left knee forward over the toes and the right heel back as a countermove. This will intensify the opening stretch in the right hip.

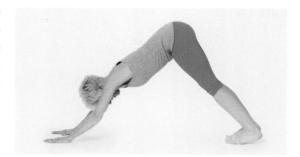

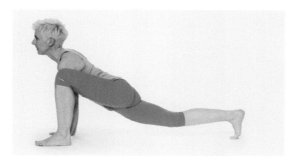

Variation 2: Add a twist towards the front leg.

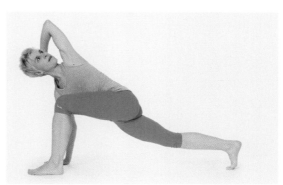

TIP

You can turn this exercise into a series by adding one element to each repetition.

ARM CIRCLE

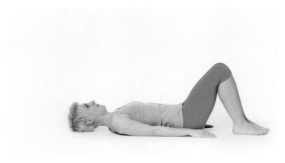

Starting position: On your back with knees bent and feet planted; arms rest alongside the body.

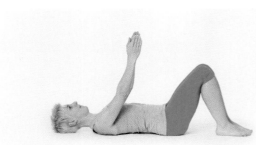

Execution: As you exhale, lift the arms off the floor and move them overhead in an arch. As you inhale, lower the arms to the sides and circle them back to the starting position.

Repeat 6-8x.

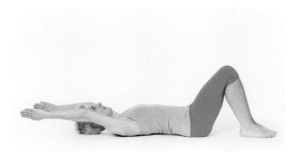
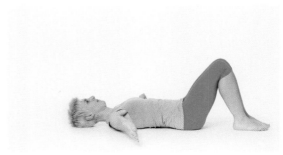

TIP

If you keep your eyes on the ceiling, you will always be able to see your fingertips. This keeps you from making the circle too big, or rather keeps the ribcage from moving.

BRIDGE

Starting position: On your back with knees bent and feet planted; knees are stacked over heels.

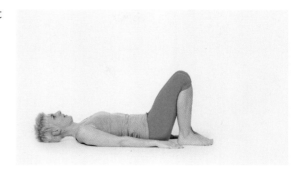

Execution: As you exhale, roll the spine up to the shoulder girdle starting with the tailbone. With the next exhalation, shift your weight to the right leg and extend the left leg to the ceiling. With each exhalation, extend the left leg forward and straighten the hip, and with each inhalation, move the leg back into the vertical position.

Repeat 6-8x per side.

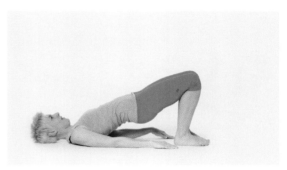

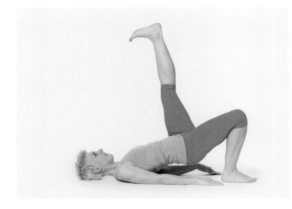

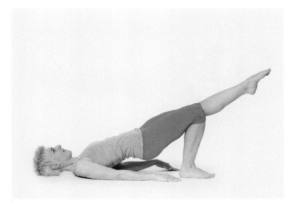

TIP
Actively press the extended arms into the floor. This will increase stability.

SINGLE-LEG STRETCH

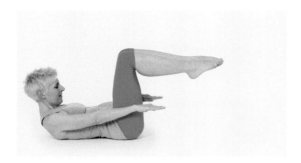

Starting position: On your back; sternum drop; knees to the body; hands alongside the body.

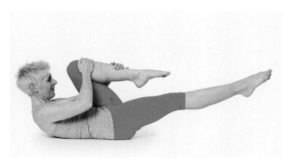

Execution: As you exhale, extend one leg forward. Hands guide the respective bent knee.

Repeat 6-8x per side.

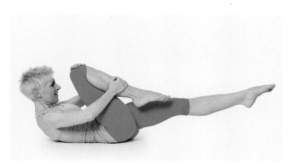

SINGLE-LEG CIRCLE

Starting position: On your back; the right leg is extended on the floor, the left leg is extended to the ceiling and slightly externally rotated; arms rest on the floor at an angle to the body, palms down.

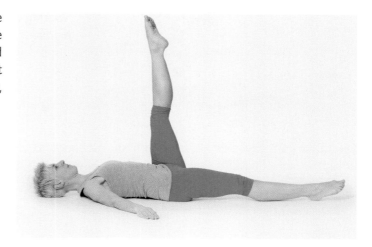

Execution: As you exhale, move the left leg in a semi-circle to the outside, and as you inhale, move it back across the midsection to the starting position.

Repeat 4-6x.

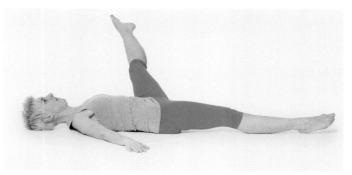

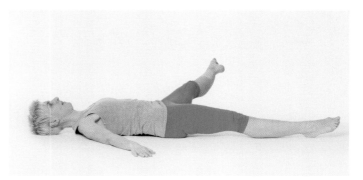

IMPORTANT

The right hip is extended and the right leg pushes out through the foot. The arms are extended to the sides and stabilize the position. The pelvis remains steady.

DART, COBRA

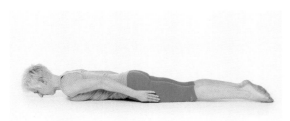

Starting position: On your stomach, arms rest alongside the body; palms face the body.

Execution: Dart. As you exhale, reach with your arms towards your feet; the thoracic spine stretches like an arrow; the upper body lifts slightly off the floor. As you exhale, lower the upper body to the floor.

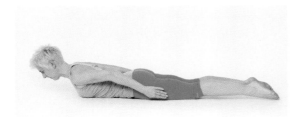 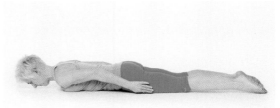

Cobra: Place the forearms on the floor in a sphinx position. As you exhale, extend the spine and push the sternum forward. The forearms pressing into the floor amplify this motion.

Repeat 4-6x.

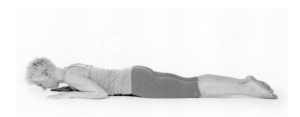 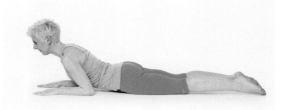

IMPORTANT
Stay centered.

ALL OF THE EXERCISES AT A GLANCE

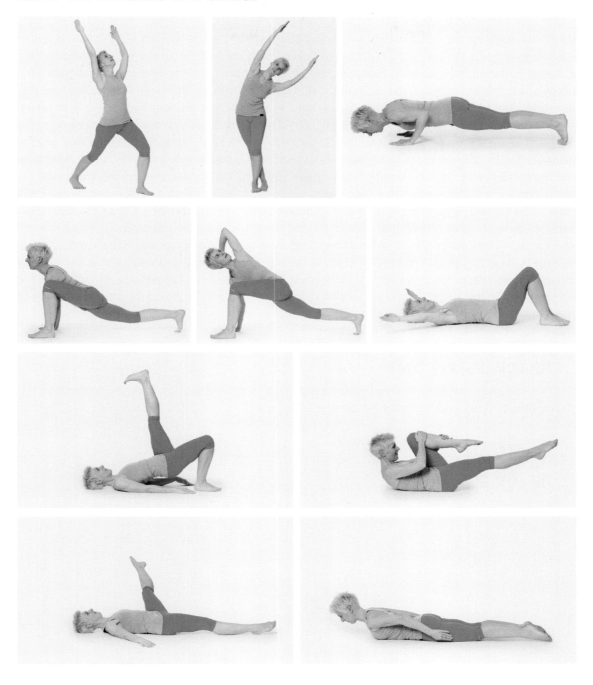

5.7   PILATES FOR RUNNERS

Man is the only mammal capable of running long distances in an upright position. More specifically, man is a born runner (see McDougal, 2010; Earls, 2014). This ability ensured our survival when we were hunter-gatherers, and even today, thousands of years later, we are still born with the same genetic programming. We still have the same body build with sturdy, elastic arches, with highly elastic Achilles tendons that store and release energy. We have strong gluteal muscles that stabilize the body and keep us from falling and are nearly tireless (see Starrett and Murphy, 2015, pg. 43ff). So why do runners continue to suffer persistent injuries? Why do runners have plantar fasciitis if the foot is designed so perfectly? And why are there Achilles tendon irritations when the Achilles tendons are elastic wonders? Why do we have knee and hip pain when our legs are supposed to be perfect springs? The answers are explicitly clear: How are feet supposed to function when they spend most of the day stuck in inappropriate footwear and don't move or aren't even noticed? How can a gluteal muscle stabilize the body when it has been completely flattened by eight hours of sitting at a desk? Healthy running over an extended period of time without any complaints only works with an accompanying exercise program. A program that includes strength and mobility training to maintain proper alignment of the feet, legs, and hips, and stabilizes the trunk during rotating movements of the pelvis and shoulder girdle. The exercises we selected focus on mobilizing the hips, ankles, and thoracic spine and on building strength and elasticity in the hip flexors and extensors to stabilize the pelvis and allow the legs to swing.

TIP FOR INSTRUCTORS

When issuing corrections, pay particular attention to the alignment of the lower extremities and include it in your explanation of the exercise.

TIP FOR STUDENTS

Supplement the workouts with ankle mobility exercises at the beginning of a unit (ankle circles, flexing and extending the feet, walking in place).

SINGLE-LEG BALANCE

Starting position: Standing with feet parallel and hip-width apart.

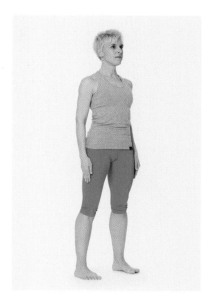

Execution: As you exhale, shift your weight to the left leg and pull the right knee into the body. Hold the right knee with one hand and extend the other arm to the side or use it to hold on to something for support. Pull the knee closer to the body several times with little pulses.

Repeat 8-10x per side.

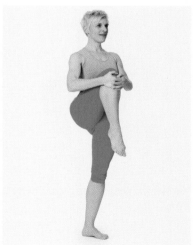

TIP
Keep the pelvis upright and allow the tailbone to pull downward as you pull the knee closer to the body.

LUNGE

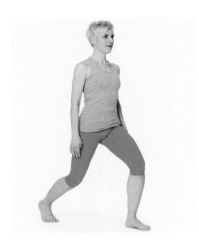

Starting position: Stand in an astride position (high lunge) with the left leg in front. Legs are parallel.

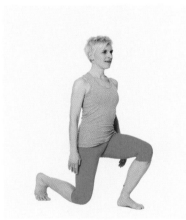
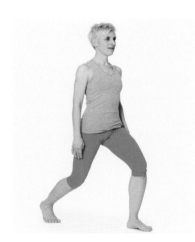

Execution: Bend the back knee towards the floor as you exhale and straighten it again as you inhale. As you do so, keep the upper body in an upright position. You can also extend the arms to the side to help with your balance.

Repeat 6-8x. After that, keep the knees bent and do small downward pulses with the back knee.

Variation: Rotate the upper body towards the closed side as you do the knee bends.

HINGE BACK AND SIT BACK

Starting position: On your knees; arms are extended in front of the body.

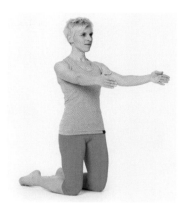

Hinge Back

Execution: As you exhale, lean back with a straight back and extended hips until you can feel a pull in the front of the thighs. Actively press the tops of the feet into the floor. As you inhale, return to the starting position.

Variation: Drop back into hip extension with a dynamic motion and then add small pulses at the end of the movement.

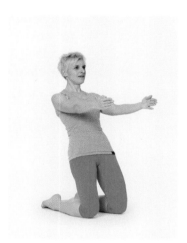
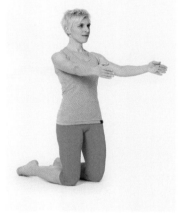

Sit Back

Execution: As you exhale, flex the hips and briefly sit back on your heels while keeping the upper body upright. As you inhale, immediately extend the hips again to return to the starting position.

Repeat 6-8x.

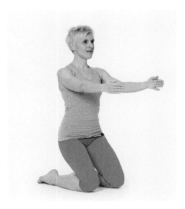
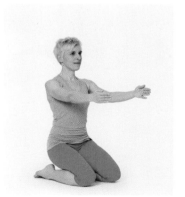

Variation: Execute the two exercises alternately with extended and flexed ankles. This will also help prevent cramping in the feet.

SHOULDER BRIDGE

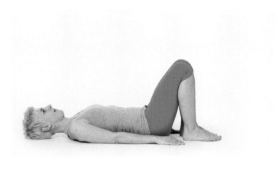

Starting position: On your back with knees bent and feet planted; knees are stacked over heels.

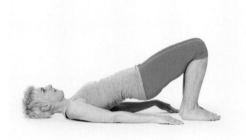

Execution: As you exhale, roll up the spine to the shoulder girdle starting with the tailbone. With the next exhalation, shift your weight to the right leg and extend the left leg to the ceiling. Now extend the left leg forward each time you exhale, and move it back into a vertical position each time you inhale.

Repeat 6-8x per side.

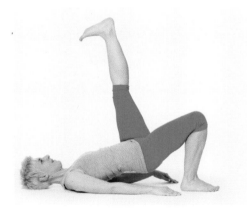

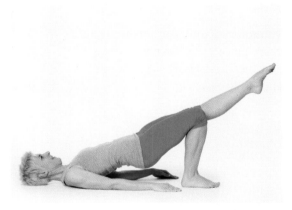

TIP
Actively press the extended arms into the floor to increase stability.

SINGLE-LEG CIRCLE

Starting position: On your back, the right leg is extended on the floor and the left leg is extended to the ceiling and slightly externally rotated. The arms rest on the floor palms down at an angle to the body.

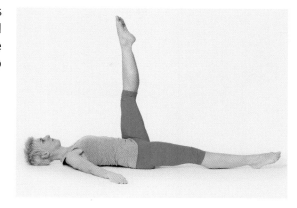

Execution: As you exhale, circle the left leg to the outside and as you inhale, move it across your midsection and back to the starting position.

Repeat 4-6x.

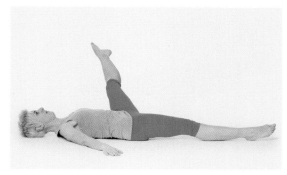

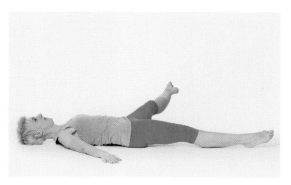

IMPORTANT
The pelvis remains steady.

SIDE KICK

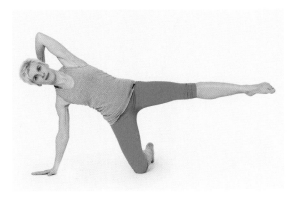

Starting position: In a side plank, the bottom knee is bent and the top leg is extended. The top hand rests against the back of the head and gently lengthens the cervical spine.

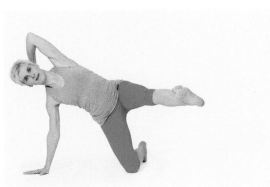

Execution: As you inhale, move the extended top leg forward, bending at the hip. The foot is flexed (dorsal flexion). As you exhale, point the foot and sweep the extended leg back into hip extension.

Repeat 6-8x.

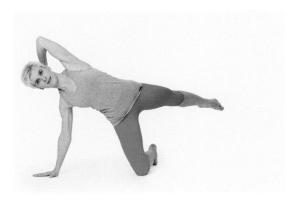

IMPORTANT

Actively press the supporting hand into the floor. This centers the shoulders and keeps the trunk steady.

DOUBLE-LEG KICK

Starting position: On your stomach, hands are folded on the tailbone, the head is turned to one side, and the knees are bent.

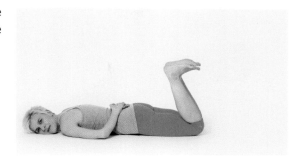

Execution: Inhale twice and kick your feet towards your pelvis 2x. As you do so, switch from flexing the feet (dorsal flexion) to pointing them (plantar flexion). As you exhale, reach with your hands towards your feet, turn the head back to the center, reach forward with the thoracic spine and reach back with your legs. As you inhale, return to the starting position and turn the head to the other side.

Repeat 6-8 x.

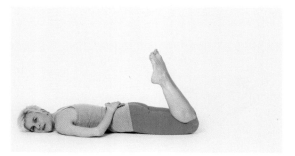

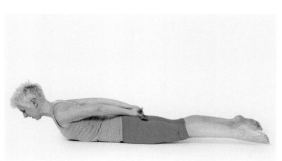

IMPORTANT
Hips remain extended during the kicks; the pelvis does not move and your backside stays down!

LEG PULL, FRONT

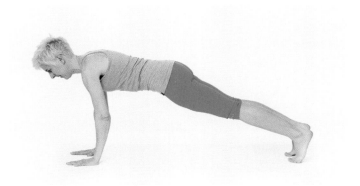

Starting position: Push-up position.

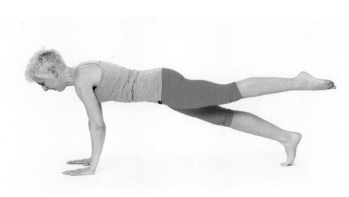

Execution: As you exhale, shift your weight to the right leg and extend the left leg back with a dynamic motion. Actively point the foot so the toes brush the floor. As you inhale, return to the starting position and switch sides.

Repeat 4-6x.

IMPORTANT

Actively push your hands into the floor and keep the shoulder girdle stable.

ALL OF THE EXERCISES AT A GLANCE

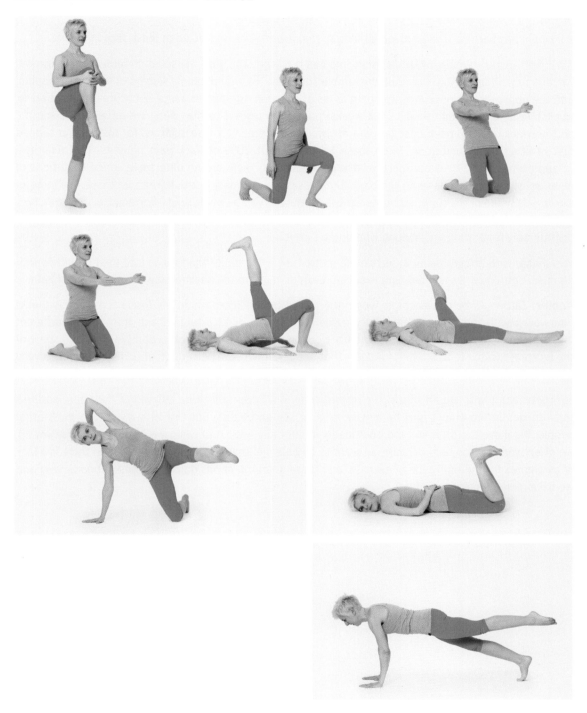

5.8 EXERCISE PROGRAM FOR A STRONG BACK

Back pain has become a widespread condition. Nearly everyone is affected at least once in his life.

Back pain comes in many different forms and can occur anywhere on the spine. In terms of localization, we refer to pain in the lower section, the lumbar spine, the lower and middle section of the thoracic spine, and the upper section or cervical spine. In terms of duration, we refer to acute, subacute (longer than six weeks), or chronic (longer than twelve weeks) pain. With respect to the cause, we differentiate specific and nonspecific back pain. Specific pain always has an organic cause such as, for instance, a slipped disk or other back conditions. These make up only about 20% of back pain patients. The majority—of approximately 80%—is nonspecific back pain, meaning there are no detectable spinal conditions or illnesses whose pain radiates to the back. The causes are disorders in the myofascial tissue, meaning in the muscle tissue or the surrounding fascial tissue. Muscles can be weak, rigid, shortened, or overstretched. Even a strong back can occasionally experience pain. However, the likelihood of recurring back pain is considerably lower than in someone who doesn't exercise.

It is similar with fascial tissue. Based on the motto "use it or lose it," the fasciae lose their resilience with non-use. Consequently, just bending over can result in injury to the back fasciae accompanied by pain.

Another cause can be the receptors within the fascial tissue. Receptors in the fascia superficialis that is interwoven with the subcutaneous fatty tissue are capable of ascertaining and transmitting different mechanical stimuli. When we don't regularly work on our self-awareness, this ability is lost and some of the receptors switch to a different function, that of nociception, the perception of pain. We become overly sensitive and even normal, easy-to-tolerate stimuli can trigger pain.

For participants with chronic back pain in particular, it is important to be relieved of their pain patterns through gentle movement and by improving their self-awareness. But this also applies to most other people: We move too little and too one-sidedly in our daily lives. And when we finally pick ourselves up, we often work out too hard because we want to be able feel that we did something. Often there is a lack of awareness for the right type of exercise, and those good intentions quickly become a boomerang and we have more pain instead of less.

It is better to get a little exercise regularly than to infrequently exercise a lot. And walk without shoes! According to Philip Beach, our feet are the sensory organs of the low back. Our feet are similarly sensitive as our hands and need unobstructed exercise to be able to do their job. That means walking barefoot on different surfaces in nature so the feet have to adapt. This will keep your feet more nimble and allows them to send the correct signals to your nervous system.

A pain-free back requires varied, diverse, appropriate, and especially regular movement and exercise.

TIPS FOR INSTRUCTORS

Work gently and consciously. Explain what is important and what should be avoided. Allow enough room for participants to reflect on the movements and become aware of their bodies. Incorporate lots of variations for the versatile and functional use of joints and tissue. Make sure the intensity of the class isn't too high. Often symptoms are delayed and participants feel good during exercise.

TIPS FOR STUDENTS

Be patient and practice regularly. Focus on your breathing and the best possible execution. In the beginning, avoid movements that cause pain. Push your limits, but don't go beyond them. Also, do those exercises you would rather skip with joy and concentration.

EXERCISE PROGRAM FOR A STRONG BACK

LOW ABS

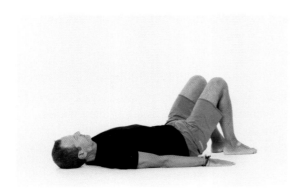

Starting position: On your back with knees bent and feet planted; arms are extended alongside the body, palms down.

Execution: Alternate lifting one leg as you exhale, and lowering it as you inhale. Repeat 3-5x per leg.

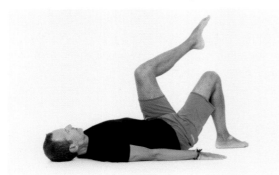 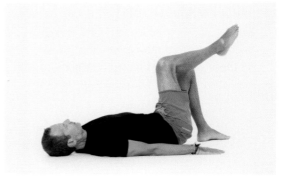

Variation: Lift both legs one after the other or simultaneously. In addition to working with parallel legs, also rotate them in and out.

TIP
Allow the calves to stay relaxed to better feel the activity of the deep hip flexors.

IMPORTANT
Keep the pelvis in a neutral position. Don't arch the back!

LEG SLIDES

Starting position: On your back with knees bent and feet planted; arms are extended alongside the body, palms down.

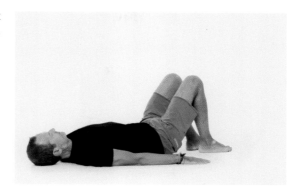

Execution: Alternate extending one leg on the floor as you inhale and bend it again as you exhale. Repeat 3-5x per leg.

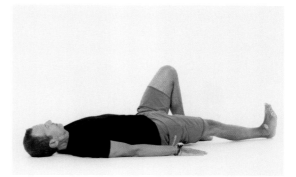

TIP

Once you've learned the basic movement, play with it. For instance, rotate the legs in and out and move them in different directions for more variety of movement.

IMPORTANT

Keep the pelvis in a neutral position. Don't arch the back!

STERNUM DROP

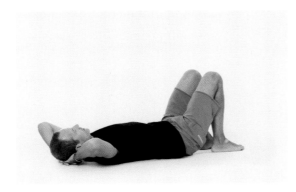

Starting position: On your back with knees bent and feet planted; both hands rest against the back of the head.

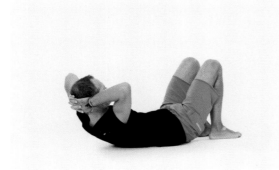

Execution: As you exhale, lift the head and shoulder blades off the floor while allowing the sternum to pull towards the pelvis. As you inhale, return to the starting position. Repeat 3-5x.

IMPORTANT

Keep the pelvis in a neutral position. Don't arch the back! Lift high enough off the floor so the upper abdominal muscles—not the neck muscles—support the head. Hands at the back of the head provide some traction but do not push!

BRIDGING

Starting position: On your back with knees bent and feet planted; arms rest alongside the body, palms down.

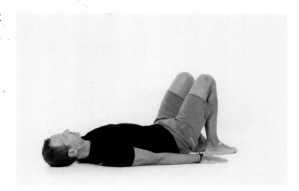

Execution: As you exhale, roll the spine up evenly starting with the pelvis and no further than the shoulder blades. Press the knees down towards the feet and consciously extend the hips without creating tension in the low back. With the next exhalation, roll back down into the starting position leading with the sternum. Imagine your warm breath melting the front of your body. Repeat 3-4x.

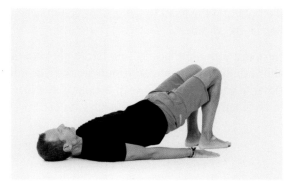

Variation: Shift the pelvis in one direction and then roll up to the right or left of the spine. Change the rhythm and range of motion.

TIP

Once you've learned the basic movement, play with it. For instance, choose different speeds and ways to roll up and down for more sensory input.

HIP ROLLS, PRETZEL STRETCH, BACK STRETCH

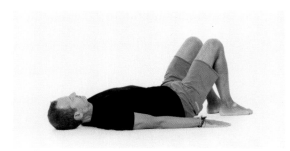

Starting position: On your back with knees bent and feet planted; arms rest alongside the body, palms down.

Execution: Extend the arms to the sides slightly below shoulder level and turn the palms over to face the ceiling. As you exhale, keep the arms and shoulder blades on the mat and rotate the legs and pelvis to the right and the head to the left. As you inhale, return to the starting position. Repeat on the left side. Repeat 3x per side.

Next, rest your right foot on your left thigh. With the left hand reach around the left leg from the outside and with the right hand reach between the legs from the inside. As you exhale, lift the legs and pull them closer to your upper body. Keep the pelvis and low back in a neutral position. Hold this position for up to three breaths, deepening the stretch with each breath. Switch sides.

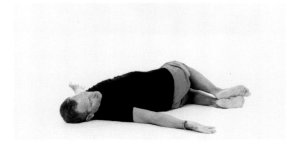

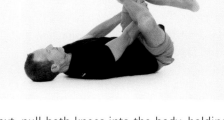

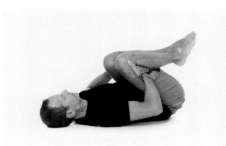

Next, pull both knees into the body, holding on to the back of the thighs or the shins. Gently pull the legs into the body to stretch the low back. Rock side to side or make small circles with your legs and hips. Repeat several times.

TIP

These exercises should help you relax and loosen up. Use only as much strength as necessary to execute the movements in a controlled manner. Take slow, even breaths. If your breathing becomes more rapid and uneven, it is a sign that you are working too hard.

SPINAL TWIST, MERMAID

Starting position: Sit in a neutral position with legs crossed; arms are extended to the sides at shoulder-level, palms down.

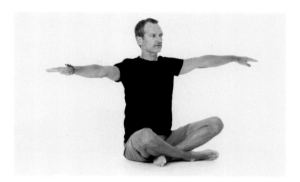

Execution: Inhale to lengthen the spine. As you exhale, turn your gaze, head, and upper body to the right. As you inhale, return to the starting position.

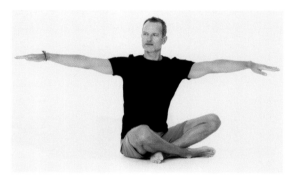

Next plant your right hand on the mat next to your hip. As you inhale, extend the left arm to the ceiling. As you exhale, bend to the right in a big arch. As you inhale, return to the starting position. Repeat 2x and then repeat on the other side.

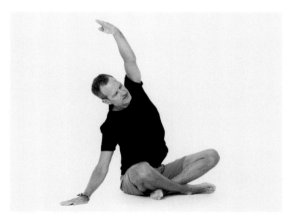

TIP

Regularly alternate legs in the cross-legged position to ensure equal effort. If you are flexible enough, you can do the spinal twist with extended legs and the mermaid with legs in a Z position.

Also practice rotating during inhalation. Rotating during inhalation facilitates axial extension and creates more space between the ribs.

DOUBLE-LEG LIFT

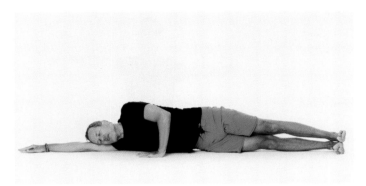

Starting position: Lie on your side in a neutral position with legs extended and closed.

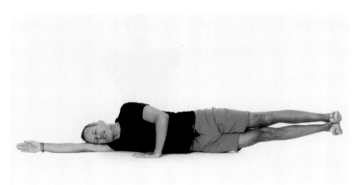

Execution: As you exhale, lift your closed legs off the mat. As you inhale, return them to the mat. Repeat 3-5x, then switch sides.

Variation: Lift the lower arm and upper body along with the legs.

TIP

In case of limited shoulder flexion, place a pillow or towel under the head and rest the lower arm on the mat in front of the body.

IMPORTANT

Keep the pelvis in a neutral position along the frontal plane. To lift the legs, lengthen the side of the body that's on the floor; to lower them, lengthen the side of the body that's off the floor. Axial extension is the key to mastering this exercise.

FOREARM SIDE PLANK

Starting position: Sit sideways on the right side of the pelvis with knees bent; the right forearm is propped on the floor at your side; elbow and shoulder are stacked.

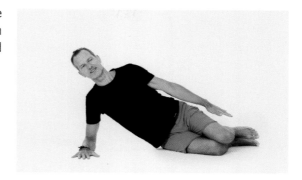

Execution: Inhale and firmly press the forearm into the mat. Create a straight line from pelvis to armpit. As you exhale, lift the pelvis off the floor. Hold for 1-2 breaths, then lower the pelvis back down to the mat as you inhale. Continue to breathe and return to the starting position. Repeat 1-3x, then switch sides.

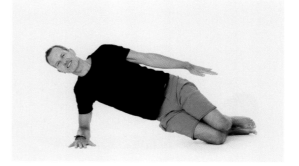

TIP

In case of weak shoulders, begin by only pressing the forearm firmly into the mat and stretching from pelvis to armpit. Once you have built up enough strength, add the pelvic lift.

IMPORTANT

Keep the pelvis in a neutral position along the frontal plane. Keep pressing the forearm into the mat to protect and stabilize the shoulder.

THE DART

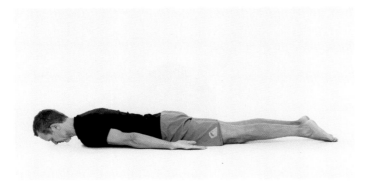

Starting position: On your stomach in a neutral position; the arms are extended on the mat alongside the body; palms face the ceiling.

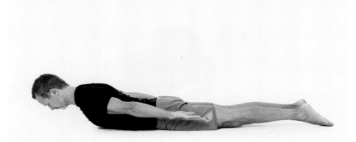

Execution: Inhale to lengthen the body. As you exhale, activate your core, reach with your arms towards your feet, push the shoulder blades towards the pelvis and lift the sternum and arms off the floor. Your upper body and head are also raised. Inhale and return to the starting position. Repeat 5-8x.

TIP

To be more comfortable, place a towel under your forehead. Tuck the toes and push the soles of the feet against an imaginary wall for more activity from deep within the body. Imagine your sternum being higher than your chin to keep the back of the neck long.

IMPORTANT

Your core is activated throughout the exercise. For more axial extension, reach with your fingertips towards your feet and reach with your head in the opposite direction. Keep your eyes on the mat and keep the back of the neck long and free of wrinkles!

STRETCHING DOG

Starting position: All-fours neutral position.

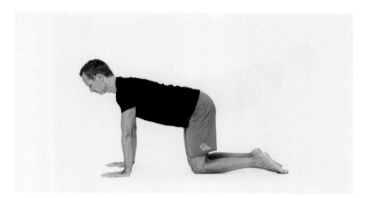

Execution: As you exhale, activate your core and extend one leg and the opposite arm parallel to the mat. Spread the fingers and toes and hold for one inhalation. As you exhale, return to the starting position. As you inhale, switch to the opposite diagonal. Repeat 3-5x per side.

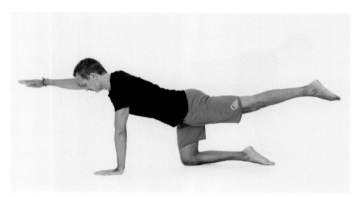

Variation: Lift arm and leg on the same side.

TIP

Begin by practicing arms and legs separately. Once you have developed sufficient stability in the pelvis and shoulder girdle, combine the arm and leg movement. Maintain contact between toes and fingertips and the mat for as long as possible. This helps you create more extension and control during lifting.

FLYING CAT

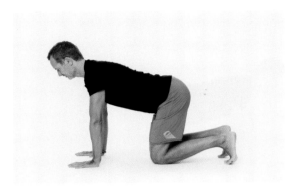

Starting position: All-fours neutral position with tucked toes.

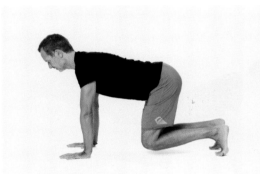

Execution: As you exhale, activate your abdominal muscles, firmly push the hands and balls of the feet into the mat and lift the lower legs a couple inches off the mat. Hold for 1-2 breaths. As you inhale, lower the lower legs back to the mat. Repeat 3-5x.

TIP

If your wrists are weak, place a rolled-up towel under the heel of your hands. For axial extension and stability, pull the sit bones back and push the crown of the head forward against an imaginary wall.

2 X 4

Starting position: Neutral standing.

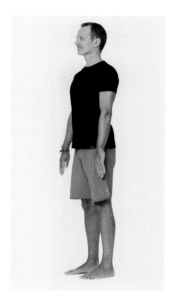

Execution: Raise the heels, bend the knees, then lower the heels back to the floor and vigorously straighten the legs, returning to the starting position. Repeat 3x, then reverse the motion sequence. Bend the knees, raise the heels, straighten the knees, lower the heels and return to the starting position. Repeat 3x.

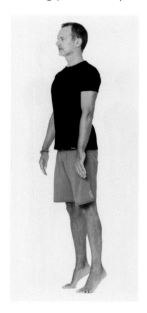 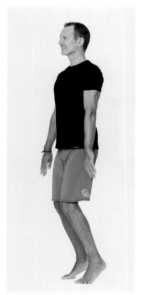 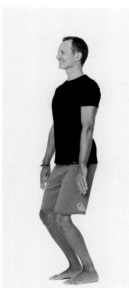 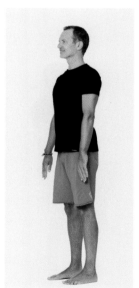

IMPORTANT

Keep the entire body as vertical as possible during the exercise and integrate the entire body into the movement.

STANDING BALANCE

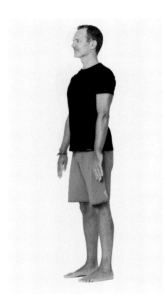

Starting position: Neutral standing.

Execution: Shift your weight to the left leg. As you exhale, press the left foot firmly into the mat, reach up through the top of the head, activate the core, and lift the right knee to approximately hip level. As you inhale, extend the arms overhead. As you exhale, lower the arms to shoulder level. As you inhale, return to the starting position. Repeat on the other side, 2-3x per side.

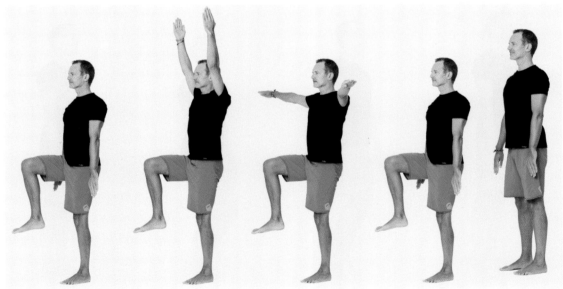

IMPORTANT

Keep the body centered by shifting your weight to the supporting leg, and keep the body as vertical as possible throughout the entire movement. Integrate the entire body into the movement.

ALL OF THE EXERCISES AT A GLANCE

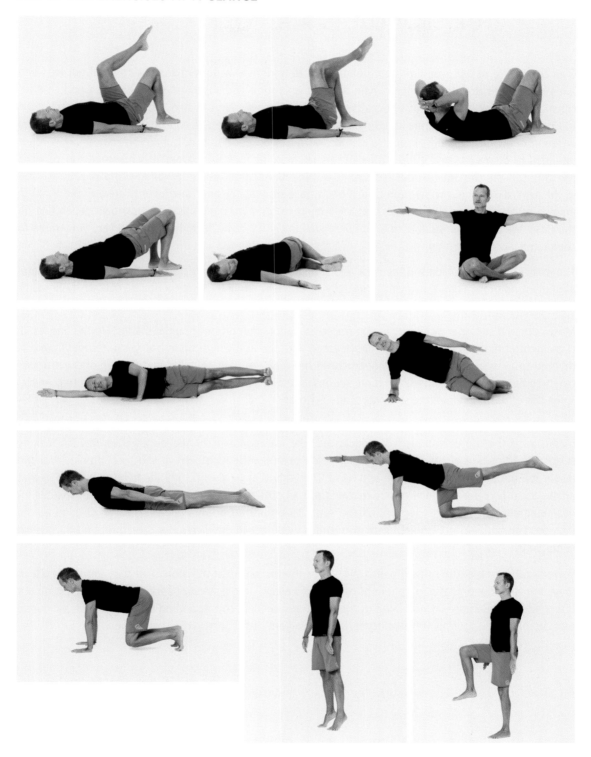

5.9 EXERCISE PROGRAM FOR SHOULDERS AND NECK

Over the course of our evolution from quadrupeds to upright-moving humans, the tasks of our legs and arms have changed a lot. Our legs' main task is locomotion and supporting our weight. Good osseous constraint is a benefit here that offers lots of freedom of movement but also sufficient stability to handle the powerful forces to be transferred. Our arms primarily help us pull and push with our hands in all different directions. While we can also support ourselves on our hands or pull up on something, it is not intended to be a sustained effort. To facilitate maximum freedom of movement while reaching, osseous constraint of the shoulder joint is reduced to a minimum and the shoulder girdle complex is connected to the axial skeleton at the sternum by just one true joint. Stability and functionality are ensured through many muscles and fascial structures that are subject to constant build-up and breakdown depending on their use. We are therefore able to adapt very well to the tasks we face, but are also very vulnerable to complaints and dysfunction.

The main causes of problems in the neck and shoulder area are due to deviations from the ideal skeletal alignment, improper breathing, and especially insufficient shoulder blade mobility, caused by heredity, work, sports, or bad habits.

Most neck and shoulder problems can be traced to dysfunction of the shoulder blades. On the one hand, it is essential that the shoulder blade move along with the arm when the arm is raised (scapulohumeral rhythm) to avoid pinching or irritating structures between the humeral head and the top of the scapula. On the other hand, some muscles that are supposed to move the shoulder blade tend to move the cervical spine out of position when the shoulder blade is frozen.

Too little or too much curvature of the thoracic spine (kyphosis) can also restrict movement of the shoulder blades with the aforementioned consequences. The misalignment of the bones does not sufficiently support the position of the shoulder girdle, which permanently lengthens or shortens muscles and can result in a misaligned cervical spine and head. The body tries to always hold the head in a position that allows us to perceive as much of our surroundings as possible. The cervical spine thus compensates for misalignments in the lower sections of the spine to ensure an optimal viewing range. Over time, the increased muscular effort required here also leads to changes in the myofascial structures and to physical complaints.

If we habitually breathe primarily into the upper thorax, we force the structures that are supposed to move our shoulder blades and upper ribs only when needed, into a steady performance state they are not intended for. This causes overloading of the structures and the corresponding symptoms such as muscle tension, painful trigger points, headaches, and movement restrictions in head and arms.

The eyes can also cause dysfunction in the neck and shoulder area. The muscles that move our eyes are closely linked to the muscles at the lower jaw and send control stimuli to the spine. A look to the right initiates a rotation. When we look up at the sky, the spine wants to bend back (extension). So we can support the movements of our spine with our eye movement, but we can also confuse our neurosensory system, for instance, when we look up while we are bending forward. In addition to muscular problems, over time this can also cause neural problems.

Our focus in choosing exercises is on the following aspects:

- Functional breathing.
- Good alignment of the spine, shoulder girdle, and head.
- The ability of the ribcage to move in all directions.
- Functional use of the abdominal muscles to promote good posture.
- Integration of the ribs.
- Shoulder blade mobility.
- Conscious use of the eyes during movements.
- Creating the scapulohumeral rhythm.

TIPS FOR INSTRUCTORS

Practicing in a seated position requires good seat height. Knees should be slightly lower than the hips and feet should be firmly planted on the floor. If this is not the case, either choose a higher seat or place a block or something similar under the student's feet. In chairs, look for a level seat that will support an upright spine. Consider initially working in front of a mirror. This will direct the focus of your awareness primarily to your vision, but it will also make it easier to align the body because our physical feeling can often send false signals.

Take your time aligning the body and breathing consciously. Both are essential to working effectively. Learning about a good and active posture and effective breathing can provide a student with much relief in everyday life.

TIPS FOR STUDENTS

Focus on the best possible execution, and in the beginning, take your time to assure proper alignment and slow and even breathing. Use a mirror to make sure that what you feel is in fact how it is supposed to be. Practice steadily and regularly. Be patient because it takes about as much time to get rid of a physical complaint as it did to create it. And don't get discouraged by less good days.

The seated exercises can also be done standing. It is easier to do the exercises while sitting down and, if necessary, you can even do them at the office.

EXERCISE PROGRAM FOR SHOUDLERS AND NECK

BREATHING, ALIGNMENT, CENTERING

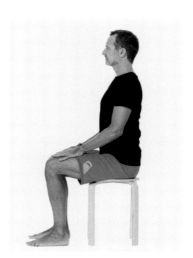

Starting position: Seated with feet planted.

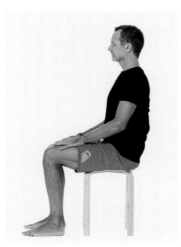
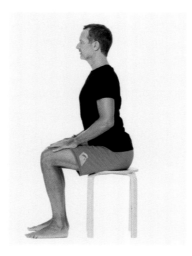

Execution: Find a neutral sitting position on your sit bones. To do so, rock the pelvis back and forth a few times and feel your weight in front, on top, and behind your sit bones. Actively push the sit bones into the seat while reaching for the ceiling with the top of the head. Inhale slowly and evenly through the nose and exhale through the mouth. Feel your breath lift and lower the abdominal wall. As you exhale, gently let the abdominal wall move towards your back and upward. Hold it in this position and breathe into the middle and lower ribcage. Emphasize breathing into the back as well as the flanks and keep the back of the neck wide and loose. As you exhale, allow the ribs to sink towards the pelvis (like a funnel or rib integration). This aligns the ribcage perfectly over the pelvis.

This is your basic position for practicing while seated.

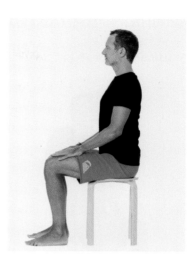

TIP

When your weight rests on your sit bones, it is impossible to sit in a slumped position. A hard chair makes it easier to feel the sit bones. To be aware of your Pilates breathing, place a towel around the middle of the back, cross the ends in front of the body and hold them in your hands. As you inhale, ease the tension when you feel your ribs press against the towel. As you exhale, pull the towel tight again.

IMPORTANT

Consciously assume this position and maintain it as you practice. If the position becomes too strenuous, take a short break and then continue practicing. Over time, you will be able to stay in this position longer.

SHOULDER RAISES AND FRONTAL PLANE SHOULDER CIRCLES

Starting position: Basic position for seated practice.

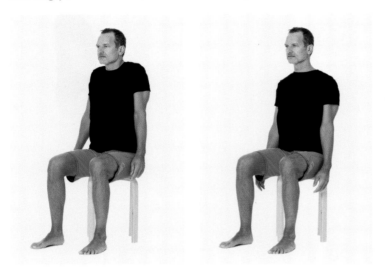

Execution: As you inhale, pull the shoulders in and up towards the ears. As you exhale, release and let the shoulders slide back into the starting position. Repeat 3-5x.

Next, circle the shoulders within the frontal plane. As you inhale, circle inward and up, as you exhale, circle outward and down. Repeat 3x, the reverse direction.

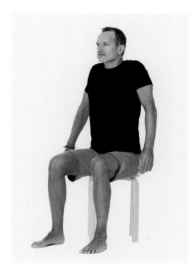 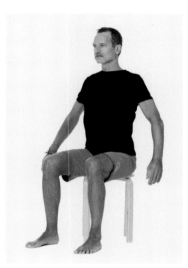 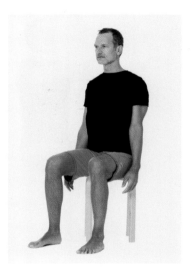

TIP

Lifting the shoulders is an active motion. Afterwards simply release and allow the shoulders to return to their natural position. At first the circles feel a little strange. Resting your hands against a wall makes the practice easier.

SCAPULA REACH

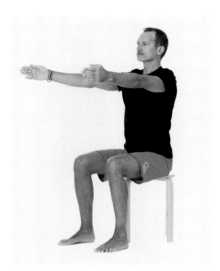

Starting position: Basic seated position with arms extended forward at shoulder level.

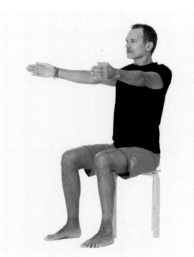

Execution: As you inhale, reach forward with your fingertips. This moves the shoulder blades away from the spine (protraction/abduction). As you exhale, pull the shoulder blades towards the spine (retraction/adduction). Repeat 3-5x.

TIP
This exercise can also be done while lying on the back or on all fours (sternum drop).

CHEST EXPANSION

Starting position: Basic seated position with arms extended and fingertips pointing to the floor and palms facing to the back.

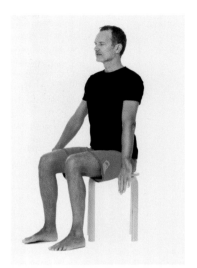

Execution: As you exhale, lengthen the spine, actively reach towards the floor with your fingertips, and with your hands, push an imaginary object back a couple inches behind the pelvis. As you inhale, return to the starting position. Keep looking straight ahead. Repeat 3-4x.

Variation: As you exhale, proceed as before, then inhale and look towards your eyebrows and push the sternum forward and up. At the same time, actively reach with your fingertips towards the floor. Release as you exhale. As you inhale, return to the starting position.

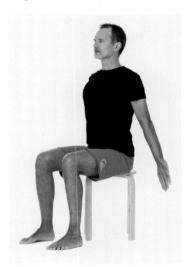

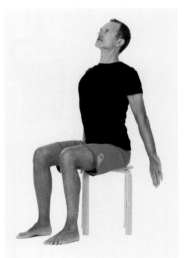

> ## TIP
> A slight internal rotation of the shoulders provides greater activation of the latissimus dorsi muscle of the back. For the variation, push the sternum forward and up, and keep the pelvis steady. During the extension you should feel like your sternum is higher than your chin. This prevents hyperextension of the neck.

SPINAL TWIST

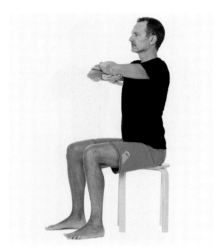

Starting position: Basic seated position; forearms are stacked in front of the chest.

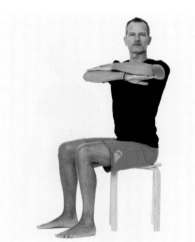

Execution: As you exhale, turn your gaze, head, and upper body to the left. As you inhale, return to the starting position. Repeat 3x per side.

IMPORTANT

Keep the pelvis steady and maintain spinal and head alignment. Keep the arms in front of the body and the gaze horizontal.

THE MERMAID

Starting position: Basic seated position; the left hand rests against the left side of the ribcage as high and close to the armpit as possible. The right arm is extended to the ceiling.

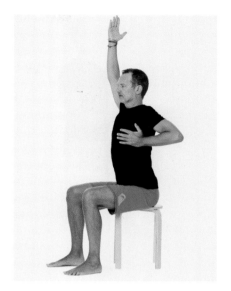

Execution: As you inhale, reach for the ceiling with your right hand and actively push the sit bones into the seat. As you exhale, create some resistance with the left hand while turning the eyes and head to the left. Then bend the spine to the left and reach overhead and to the left with the right arm in a big arch. Repeat 2-3x. Then remove the left hand from the ribcage, reflect, and repeat the same sequence on the other side.

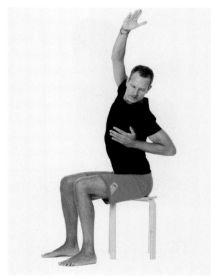

TIP

By holding your hand against the ribcage during the side bend, you are primarily opening the area between the ribs. If you want to put more emphasis on the area between ribcage and pelvis, work without holding your hands against your ribs. Execute the movement with small rotations to the front and the back to reach different parts of the trunk musculature.

THE WAITER

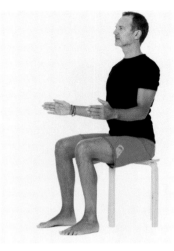

Starting position: Sit as before; arms are at your sides with elbows bent at a 90-degree angle. Fingertips point forward.

Execution: As you exhale, rotate the arms out. As you inhale, return to the starting position. Repeat 3-5x.

Variation: Add a spinal extension.

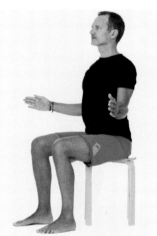 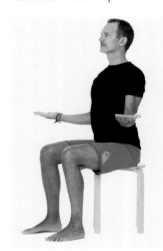 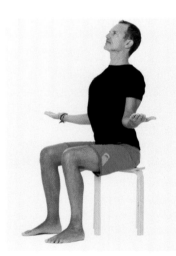

TIP

Play with the position of the palms during the movement (facing the floor, the ceiling, each other) for more variety of movement.

IMPORTANT

Hold the elbows slightly in front of the shoulders. To actively keep the arms tucked against the body without pressing the elbows into your sides, imagine holding a rolled-up newspaper under your armpit. Maintain neutral alignment throughout the arm movement.

ALL OF THE EXERCISES AT A GLANCE

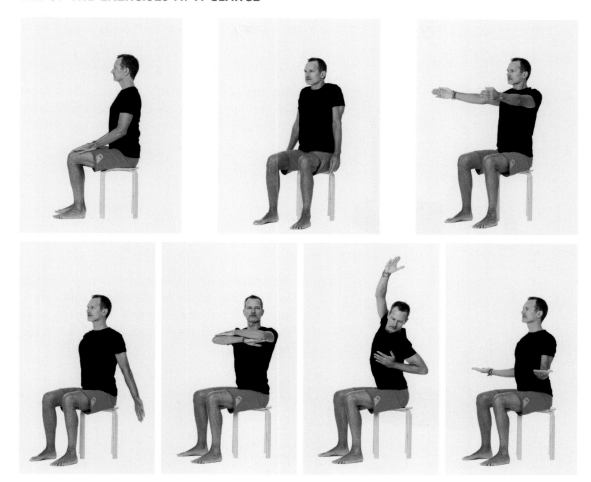

EXERCISES IN ALTERNATIVE BASIC POSITIONS

SCAPULA REACH

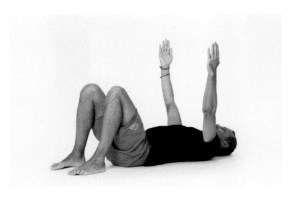

Starting position: Neutral supine position; knees are bent or extended; the arms are extended to the ceiling over the shoulders, palms face each other.

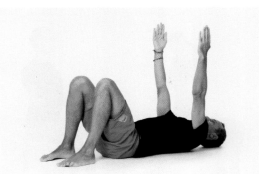

Execution: As you inhale, reach with your fingertips for the ceiling. As you exhale, return to the starting position. Initiate the movement with the shoulder blades and feel them glide across the ribcage. Repeat 3-5x.

TIP
Play with the arm alignment during the movement (internal rotation, external rotation) for more variety of movement. Bend and straighten the elbows to activate the entire movement chain with the arms.

TELESCOPING ARM, BOOK OPENING

Starting position: On your side; legs are in a 90/90-degree position; the head is cushioned and the arms are extended forward and stacked in front of the sternum.

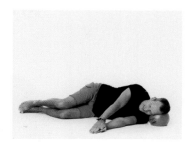

Execution: As you inhale, reach forward with the top arm. As you exhale, pull it back again. As you do so, roll the spine forward and back and move the shoulder blades along the ribcage. Repeat 2-3x.

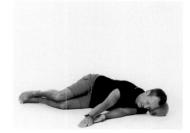 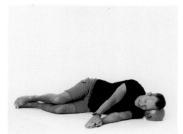

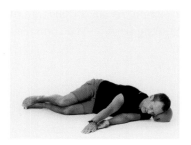 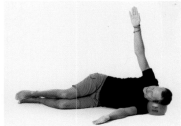 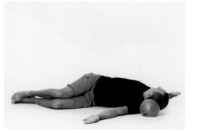

Next, as you inhale, reach forward again with the top arm. As you exhale, release the top arm and start to roll onto your back. Track the top arm with your eyes. When you are done rotating the spine, inhale, reach with both arms towards the opposite walls, and as you exhale, return to the starting position. Repeat 2-3x and switch sides.

TIP

Hold a ball between your hands during the telescoping arm movement to emphasize the gliding motion. During the book opening, consciously press the bottom arm into the mat and lengthen it through the fingertips. This will create more space between the shoulder blades and increases rotation.

SIDE BEND IN SIDE PLANK

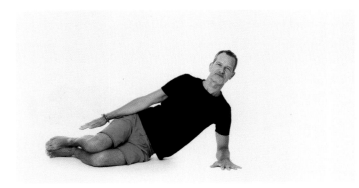

Starting position: Side plank with knees bent; the top hand rests on the upper iliac crest.

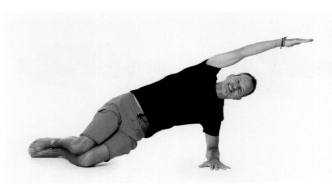

Execution: As you inhale, firmly push the forearm into the mat and the pelvis towards the feet. Lift the trunk towards the ceiling in a long line or into an even arch and move the top arm up and over the head in a big circular motion. As you exhale, return to the starting position in a controlled motion.

TIP

As you lift the trunk, externally rotate the supporting arm and internally rotate it as you lower back down. Turn your gaze and head towards the floor as you lift the trunk, and look towards the pelvis or feet as you lower back down.

IMPORTANT

Keep the body in the frontal plane.

COBRA

Starting position: On your stomach; arms are extended forward at least shoulder-width apart.

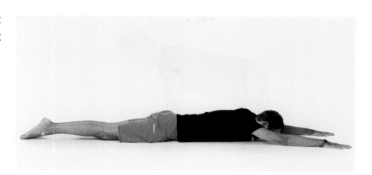

Execution: As you exhale, activate the core, lengthen through the legs, look towards your eyebrows, push the sternum forward, lift the upper body, and simultaneously pull the elbows under the shoulders. Hold for several breaths, then lengthen the body as you inhale; as you exhale, look to your cheek bones and return to the starting position. Repeat 2-3x.

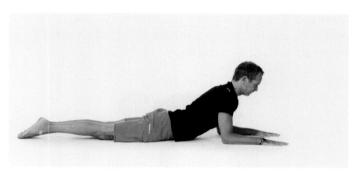

TIP

Firmly push the arms into the mat and lengthen the body from the sternum to the feet. For more activation of the deep structures, tuck the toes and push the soles of the feet against an imaginary wall.

STERNUM DROP, THREAD THE NEEDLE

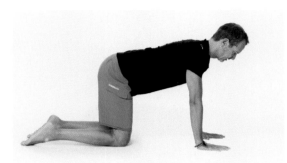

Starting position: Neutral all-fours position.

Execution: As you exhale, push the sternum up towards the ceiling and create space between the shoulder blades. As you inhale, lower the sternum towards the floor and squeeze the shoulder blades together tightly at the back. Repeat 3-5x.

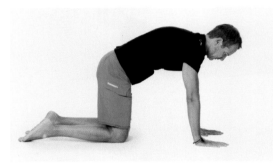

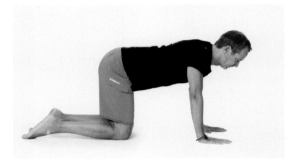

Variation: Reverse your breathing pattern.

Then slide the left hand under the right arm with the palm facing the ceiling. As you do so, bend the right elbow for a clean rotation. As you inhale, return to the starting position. Repeat 3x, then switch sides.

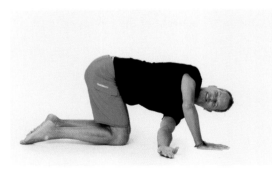

TIP

Actively press the hands into the mat for better awareness of your shoulder blades. Begin to thread the needle with your eyes and shift them to where you wish to rotate. Pull the sit bones back for axial length and stability.

REFLECTION

Starting position: Standing

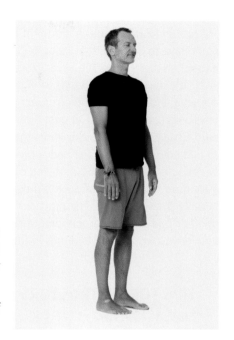

Execution: Stand tall in neutral alignment and reflect on the movements. How do your shoulders and neck feel? Is your head floating? Do you carry it proudly? How do you perceive your erect posture and breath?

Now take a few steps across the room and become aware of yourself in motion.

TIP

Do not skip this part! Every day is different and gives you the opportunity to perceive yourself anew and develop body awareness.

5.10   FIT FOR LIFE

For Joseph Pilates, it was a matter of course: The daily practice of his exercises. He made no excuses. We don't have to be quite that strict. But 2-3 practice units per week are necessary to counteract the body's natural changes (read the Silver Mover section even if you are still young) and maintain a basic fitness level. It's not about engaging in high-performance sports but about integrating Pilates principles into everyday life, about shedding inaccurate movement patterns and programming new, economical, and physiological processes. Frequent problems such as muscle tension, restriction of motion, and back or joint pain, usually improve quickly with regular exercise. The practice should be in line with the fitness level but should not be too easy. The body only reacts when the stimulus is strong enough. Getting out of breath or sweating is not bad. Get out of your comfort zone and into the movement zone. It's fine to use all kinds of assistance to get through such a program. Assistance can be in the form of a routine, a progression that initially stays the same. The practicing person quickly notices the differences in execution, progress, and good or bad days. A routine progression gives you parameters that allow you to measure your progress and let you focus on new details in the exercises or in the body.

TIPS FOR INSTRUCTORS

Take as much care of yourself as you do of your participants. This includes your own regular practice. An instructor's body is his biggest capital. It is a role model, example, and walking advertising all the way into old age.

ONE HUNDRED

Starting position: On your back with knees bent and feet planted. Head and shoulder girdle are rolled up (sternum drop); arms are extended alongside the body; palms down.

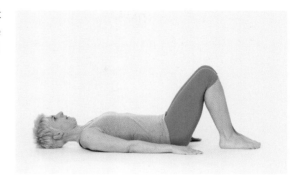

Execution: Roll up head and shoulders. Take 5 quick breaths through the nose and exhale 5x through the nose or mouth while vigorously pumping the arms up and down. Pump up to 100x, then roll head, arms, and legs back down to the mat.

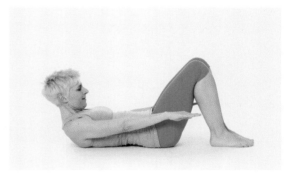

TIP

Build up your breathing in stages: first inhale 2x and exhale 2x, then 3x, 4x, etc.

ROLL UP

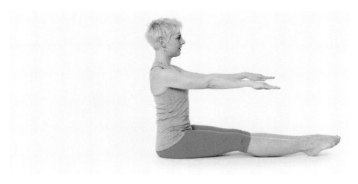

Starting position: Seated with legs extended.

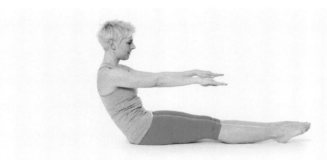

Execution: Working with the breath, roll the spine down into a supine position starting at the tailbone.

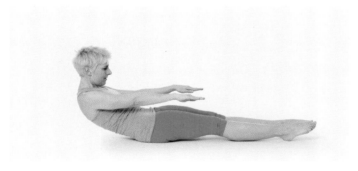

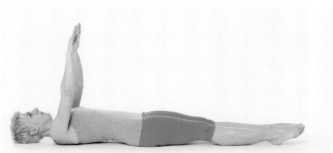

The arms accompany the movement until the fingertips point to the ceiling.

As you exhale, start with the head and roll the spine back up until the upper body is rounded over the legs. The pelvis remains upright. Then roll back down from this position.

Repeat 4-6x.

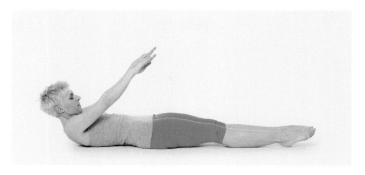

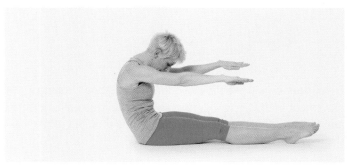

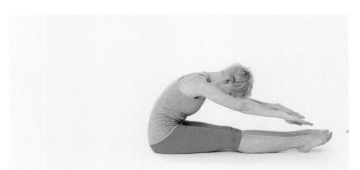

IMPORTANT

The motion sequence should be fluid and even.

TIP

Hands and feet reach forward.

ROLL OVER

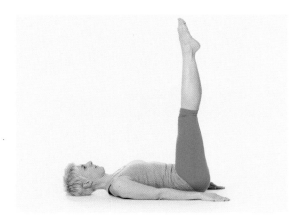

Starting position: On your back; legs are closed and extended to the ceiling; arms are extended alongside the body.

Execution: As you exhale, move the legs overhead, rolling up the spine to the shoulder girdle. Initiate the movement with the pelvic floor and let the toes push up and back. The arms press down into the floor and forward. Once you have landed on the shoulder girdle, flex the feet (dorsal flexion) and slightly open the legs.

With your next exhalation, roll back into the starting position vertebrae by vertebrae. Pressing the arms into the floor and the head's counteraction support a controlled rolling back.

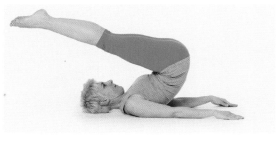

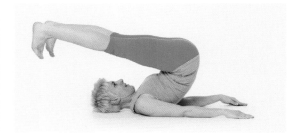

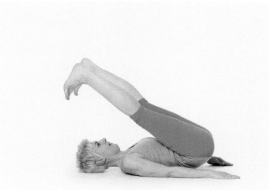

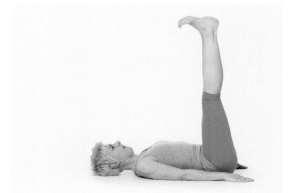

Once you have landed on the sacrum, extend the feet again and start over.

Repeat 6-8x.

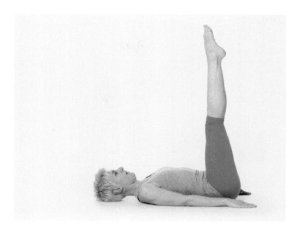

IMPORTANT

Only roll up as far as the shoulder girdle, meaning up to the shoulder blades. The cervical spine remains long.

PILATES

BRIDGE

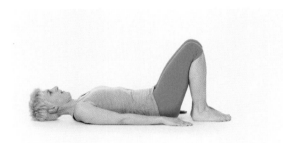

Starting position: On your back in a neutral position with knees bent and feet planted; knees are stacked over heels; legs are parallel and hip-width apart; arms rest alongside the body.

Execution: As you exhale, roll up the spine starting at the tailbone and up to the shoulder girdle. With your next exhalation, shift your weight to the right leg and extend the left leg to the ceiling. Each time you exhale, extend the left leg forward, and as you inhale, move the leg back into a vertical position, keeping the foot flexed (dorsal extension).

Repeat 6-8x.

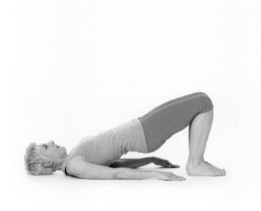

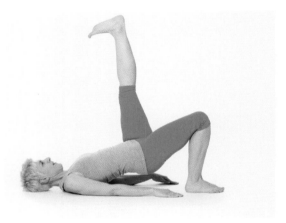

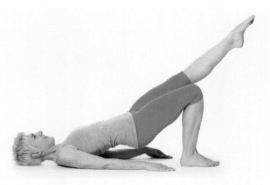

TIP
Actively press the extended arms into the floor to increase stability.

SIDE KICK

Starting position: In a side-lying position, the bottom leg is bent and the top leg is extended and raised to hip-level.

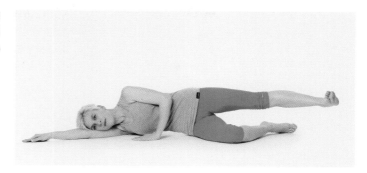

Execution: As you inhale, bend the hip and move the leg forward. The foot is in dorsal extension. As you exhale, extend the hip and move the top leg back with toes pointed.

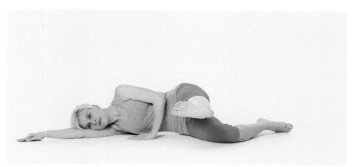

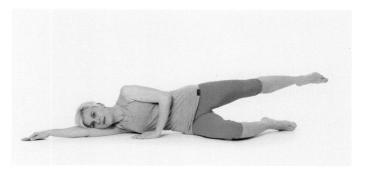

IMPORTANT
The pelvis remains steady. Remember the air cushion under the waist.

SAW

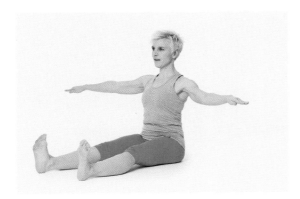

Starting position: Seated position with legs extended and shoulder-width apart; feet are in dorsal extension; arms are laterally extended.

Execution: As you inhale, rotate the spine to the left around its vertical axis. As you exhale, bend the spine to reach towards the left foot with the right hand. As you inhale, roll up and exhale back to the starting position.

Repeat 4-6 x.

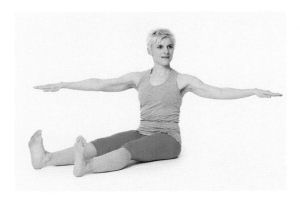
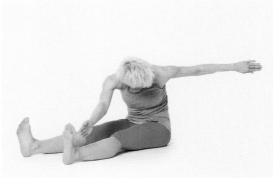

IMPORTANT

The pelvis remains steady and both sit bones maintain contact with the floor.

STRETCHING DOG

Starting position: On all fours.

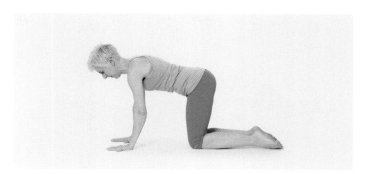

Execution: As you exhale, shift your weight to the right hand and left leg; next, let the left arm and right leg first slide across the floor and then lift the fully extended arm and leg off the floor. As you inhale, return to the starting position.

Repeat 4-6x, alternating sides.

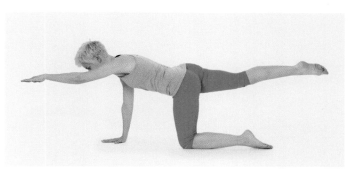

TIP FOR INSTRUCTORS

Emphasize extension during verbal instructions to keep the shoulder and pelvic girdles parallel to the floor and avoid arching the back.

SWIMMING

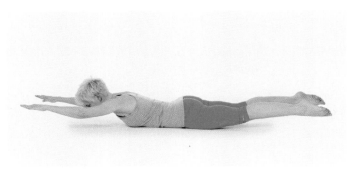

Starting position: On your stomach; arms and legs are extended and raised.

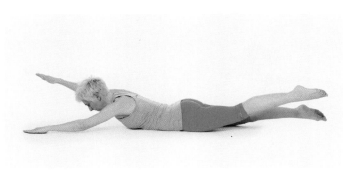

Execution: Paddle opposing arms and legs on a diagonal, keeping an even pace. Breathe slowly and evenly and complete 5 strokes during every inhalation and exhalation phase.

IMPORTANT
Stay centered!

ALL OF THE EXERCISES AT A GLANCE

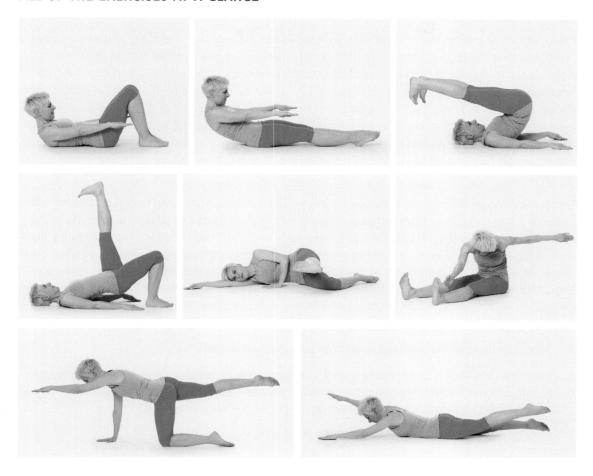

5.11   FASCIA PILATES

Fascia are all of the fibrous and collagen connective-tissue structures, including tendons, ligaments, capsules, and muscles. The significance of the fascia was long underestimated. But international fascia research and its current insights have made it clear that the collagen network plays an important role in force transmission and provides an important basis for flexibility, elasticity, and physical performance. We are not at all talking about an insignificant tissue that merely serves as a covering for something more important like, for instance, muscles. Fascia have enormous influence on the muscles, locomotion, posture, and pain perception. Fascia permeate the entire body like a three-dimensional network, and, depending on the amount of loading and demands placed on them, can be thick and strong or fine and delicate.

They are located at different depths inside the body and envelop muscles, cling to organs, and are linked throughout the body. This creates a fascia bodysuit that lends the body its silhouette, provides support, ensures the smooth gliding of structures within the body, and keeps them flexible. Furthermore, the body-wide collagen network is equipped with many receptors and thus is an important sensory organ that also affects pain perception. In short, fascia must be taken into account in physical fitness and in recreational and competitive sports training. The Pilates practice already includes many elements of fascia training. The ideal fascia workout is based on the four fascia fitness principles (see *Journal of Bodywork & Movement Therapies* [2012], 1-13):

1. Rebound elasticity: the elastic rebound with preparatory countermotion.

2. Slow and dynamic rotations: the intended movements are rather long-chain in different directions or with different vectors. Slow stretches are also described as melting into the movement. Dynamic stretches are characterized by small pulses at the end of the range of motion.

3. Proprioceptive refinement: refined feeling focusing on body awareness.

4. Hydration of the matrix: working the tissue with massage rollers and balls.

We limited our selection of exercises to principles 1-3 and left out the principle of matrix hydration. The focus is thus on the active exercises and the unit can be completed without supplementary material.

TIPS FOR INSTRUCTORS

In the beginning, the new training stimuli via the fascia fitness principles can be very strenuous (rebound elasticity) or unfamiliar (proprioceptive refinement). Choose short sequences and allow enough freedom for your personal perception and execution. We therefore forgo listing a recommended number of repetitions for some of the exercises. Most of the time we don't make detailed breathing suggestions either. It is more important that the participants are able to coordinate their breathing with the respective movement. Of course this presupposes that the participants are familiar with the breathing principle. We also recommend that the modified exercises first be learned in their original form so the fascia fitness principles are met with a sound foundation. Otherwise there is the danger of muscle strains or similar injuries, particularly in the area of rebound elasticity.

TIPS FOR STUDENTS

Admittedly, some of the exercises look like they harken back to the days of Father Jahn, the father of German gymnastics, while others seem rather strange. Keep an open mind, listen to your body, and let it experience something new and different.

KNEE BOUNCES

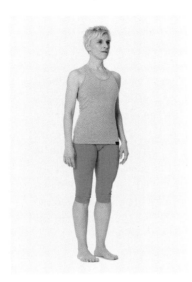

Starting position: Standing; feet are planted hip-width apart and parallel.

Execution: Bounce rhythmically and evenly in the knees. Also do so with the hips rotated in and out.

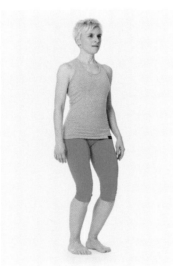
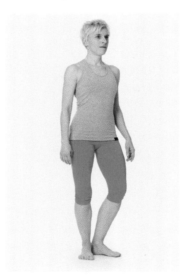
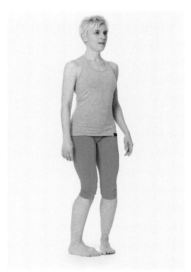

Variation: Lift the feet higher off the floor (double bounce) with every other bounce so every second bounce becomes a jump. The motion originates in the feet. The sole of the foot (plantar fascia) tightens during the downward movement and relaxes during the opposing upward movement.

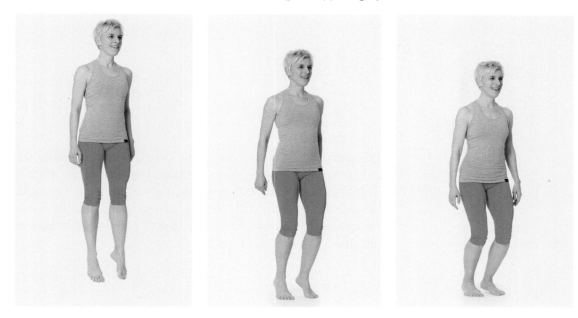

Typical fascia Pilates: Bouncing movements and different directions and vectors.

IMPORTANT
Watch the alignment, particularly of knees and feet.

FRONT SWING

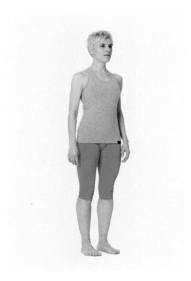

Starting position: Standing; feet are planted hip-width apart and parallel.

Execution: As you inhale, extend the sternum and the arms to the ceiling and press the feet into the floor. The front of the body is preloaded like a bow. As you exhale, release the tension to allow the dynamic forward swing of the upper body and arms to follow. The gaze shifts towards the abdominal wall and the pelvis remains upright.

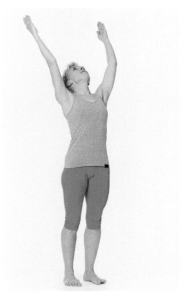
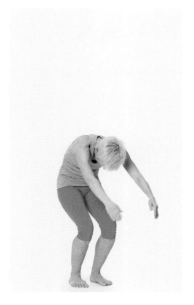
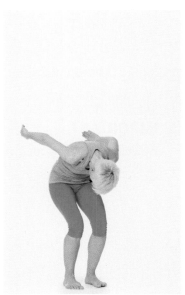

Typical fascia Pilates: Build and release body tension (see tensegrity in the alignment section); preparatory countermovement followed by the elastic rebound (rebound elasticity).

IMPORTANT

This very dynamic countermovement should initially be performed slowly and with guidance. The Pilates principle of centering has been learned beforehand so the pelvis and lumbar spine will be protected during the elastic rebound.

MAD CAT VARIATION

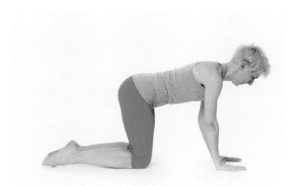

Starting position: On all fours.

Execution: As you exhale, bend the spine by pressing the hands and feet into the floor and rounding the spine into a big arch. With your next exhalation, straighten the spine and separate the tailbone and the top of the head. Hands and knees pull towards each other. Repeat several times, alternating positions.

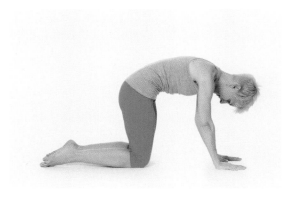

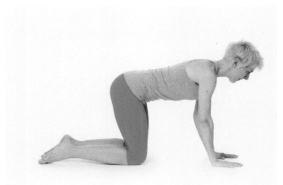

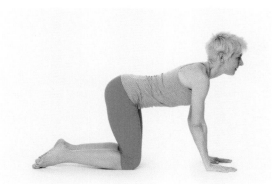

Laterally pull head and tailbone towards each other in lateral flexion (side bend) while keeping the spine parallel to the floor.

Then link all directions, creating a kind of circle. Change directions. Then create different connections like a billiard ball that rolls from cushion to cushion in slow motion, always using different angles as it ricochets.

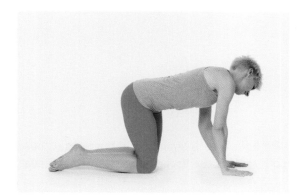 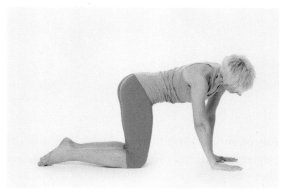

Typical fascia Pilates: Independent exploration of the different directions and the spine's capabilities and a continuous comparison between the way the new directions feel in comparison to the previous movements (proprioceptive refinement).

TIP

Use images (e.g., billiard ball [see exercise description] or The trunk is inside a tube or a barrel and the costal arches should glide along the inside of the tube in a circular motion).

UP STRETCH

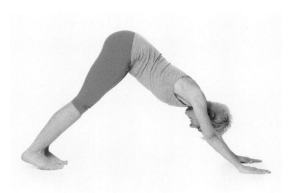

Starting position: From all-fours position into up-stretch position.

Execution: Push the right heel towards the floor 2x. The right knee is straight and the right sit bone pushes towards the ceiling. The left knee is bent and pulls towards the floor. The pelvis rotates. Repeat, alternating sides.

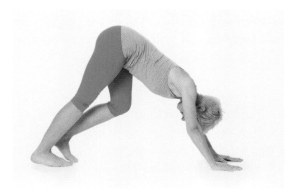
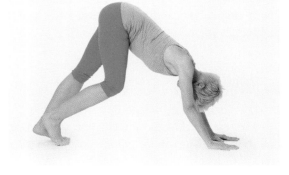

Variation: Modify by rotating the hips in and out.

Typical fascia Pilates: Pulsing movements and different directions and vectors.

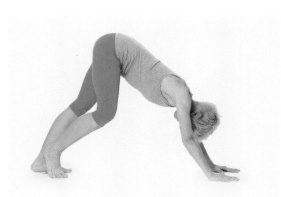

TWIST

Starting position: Cross-legged seat; arms are laterally extended; palms face the floor.

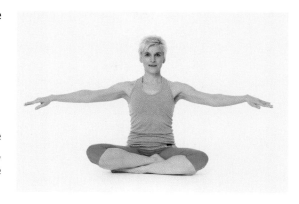

Execution: As you inhale, rotate the trunk to the right to preload it like a spring. As you exhale, release the tension so the trunk can rebound in the opposite direction. Repeat 6-8x, then switch sides.

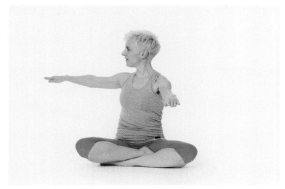
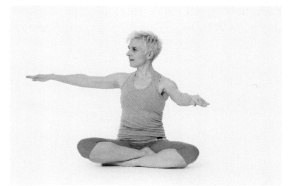

Typical fascia Pilates: Pulsing movements; building and releasing body tension (see tensegrity in the alignment section); preparatory countermovement followed by an elastic rebound.

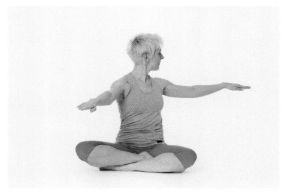

TIP

This exercise is even more dynamic when it is supplemented with the dynamic stretching principle. To do so, pre-tighten first and then release tension during the rotation, and add 2-3 pulses at the end of the rotation. Adjust your breathing rhythm accordingly (e.g., inhale and pre-tighten 1x, then exhale 2-3x for the pulses at the end of the movement).

SAW

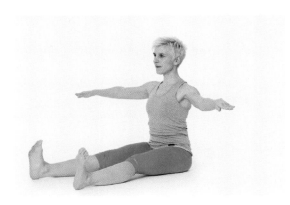

Starting position: Seated with legs extended and slightly apart; feet are flexed.

Execution: As you inhale, sit up tall, and as you exhale, reach with your right hand towards your left foot and pulse 2-3x. As you inhale, sit up again and switch sides.

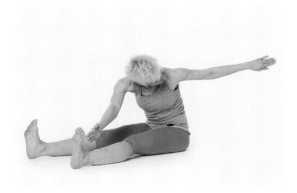

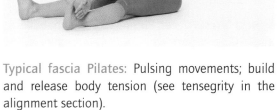

Typical fascia Pilates: Pulsing movements; build and release body tension (see tensegrity in the alignment section).

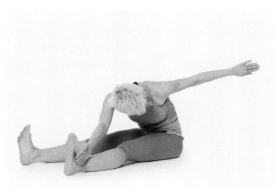

IMPORTANT

The pelvis remains steady in spite of the dynamic movements; both sit bones maintain contact with the floor.

BOUNCE DOWN

Starting position: Seated with legs extended.

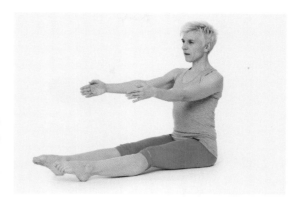

Execution: Tilt the pelvis (curl down) and roll down the spine to approximately the sacrum. Then pulse a few times, lengthening the spine a little more with each pulse. Then roll down a little further and pulse there. Gradually roll down more and pulse until you are in a supine position.

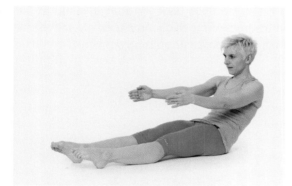
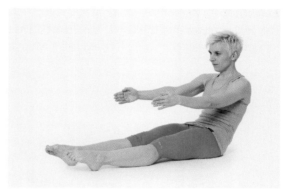

Typical fascia Pilates: Pulsing movements; build and release body tension (see tensegrity in the alignment section).

TIP
Of course it is physiologically impossible to pulse vertebrae by vertebrae. But imagining that each vertebra is its own level where pulses take place facilitates segmental control and movement.

SIDE-LYING LEG WHIP

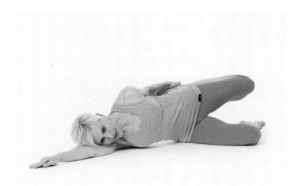

Starting position: On your side; the bottom knee is bent; grip the top ankle.

Execution: As you inhale, pre-tighten the top leg by pushing the thigh back and straightening the hip. The ankle presses into the hand. This creates tension in the front of the thigh. As you exhale, release the tension so the leg can swing forward like a whip and then spring back into starting position.

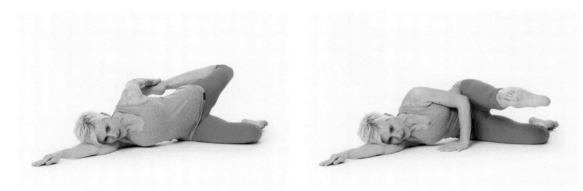

Typical fascia Pilates: Build and release body tension (see tensegrity in the alignment section).

IMPORTANT
Prerequisite is the correct execution of the side kick exercise.

SIDE TO SIDE

Starting position: On your back; arms and legs are extended.

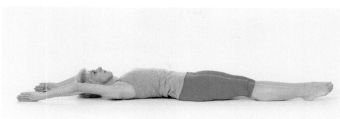

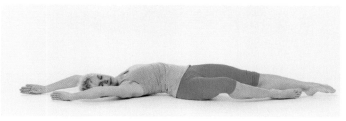

Execution: Build up tension in the left flank by pulling the left leg and left arm up, or rather down, lengthening the left flank. The right side of the body (i.e., left arm and leg) is bent. Release the tension again. Repeat several times to emphasize the link between pulling on the left side and the resulting bend in the right side.

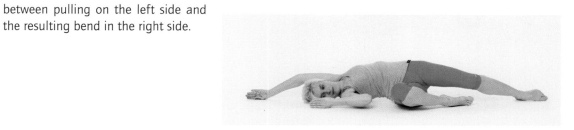

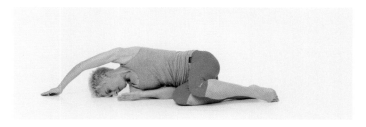

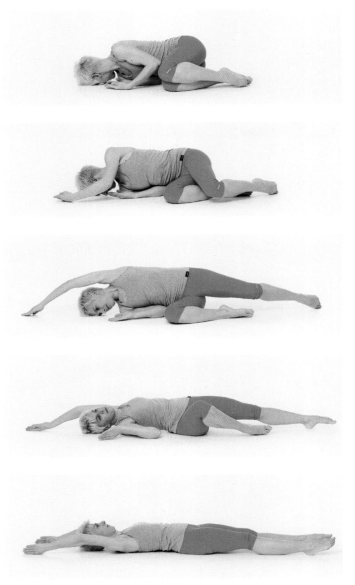

The more tension that is created on the left side, the more the right side glides into an embryo-like posture.

Now reverse the movement. By opening up the left side, the body glides back into the starting position.

Typical fascia Pilates: Exploration of movement approach, cause and effect of movement (proprioceptive refinement).

TIP

Maintain constant contact between arms and hands, legs and feet, and the floor.

ALL OF THE EXERCISES AT A GLANCE

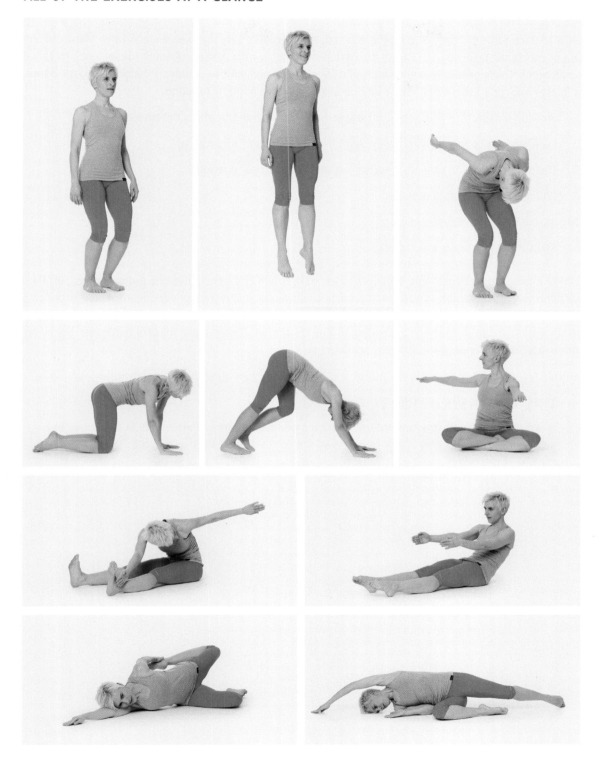

5.12   PILATES WITH SMALL IMPLEMENTS

Next to the traditional mat exercises there are countless ways to vary the exercise repertoire. Many of them are in this book. One way to change up Pilates exercises is with the use of small implements, so-called small props. These generally include balls of different sizes and various degrees of hardness, elastic bands, a Pilates ring, or a foam roller. These small implements have multiple functions:

1.   Individual aspects of exercises can be specifically augmented to refine the exercises.

2.   Exercises can be made easier (regression) or more difficult (progression).

3.   The modifications to familiar exercises expand the exercise repertoire.

4.   Change the focus of an exercise.

5.   Introduce studio equipment.

6.   Keep classes versatile and exciting.

Unlike Pilates studio equipment, small props are inexpensive and easy to use in a group setting. Different facilities (e.g., sports clubs, fitness studios, etc.) usually already have a lot of equipment. And if they don't, there are small props, meaning they are of a size that allows the instructor to take them to different locations. Important for facilities: It is easy to find a suitable storage place for new purchases. Below are three exercise sequences with different small props.

TIPS FOR INSTRUCTORS

It is not necessary to structure the entire class around small props. Particularly in the beginning, it is enough to offer only a few exercises so the focus doesn't shift so much to the implement instead of the body.

5.12.1 THE PILATES BALL

In recent years, many Pilates instructors have added the Pilates ball to their repertoire. Its low cost and its versatility due to its different sizes (18-26 cm diameter) make it very versatile and popular with both instructors and students.

By inflating it to different levels, it can lend support for exercises or make them more difficult. It can be used for resistance to better activate the body, for balance, as a pillow, or to change the movement path.

TIPS FOR STUDENTS

Begin by using the Pilates ball so it helps you to better understand the exercises and for support. Once you have more experience with the exercises and the handling of the ball, you can also use it as a challenge.

EXERCISE PROGRAM WITH THE PILATES BALL

PELVIC CLOCK, LOW ABS

Starting position: On your back with knees bent; the ball is placed under the sacrum.

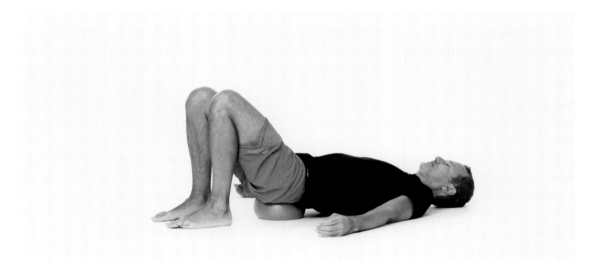

Execution: Breathe slowly and steadily while circling the pelvis several times on the ball, first clockwise then counterclockwise. When circling counterclockwise, gradually make the circles smaller until the pelvis just rests on the ball.

Next alternately lift one leg off the floor and lower it. Lift as you exhale and lower as you inhale. Repeat 3-5x per leg.

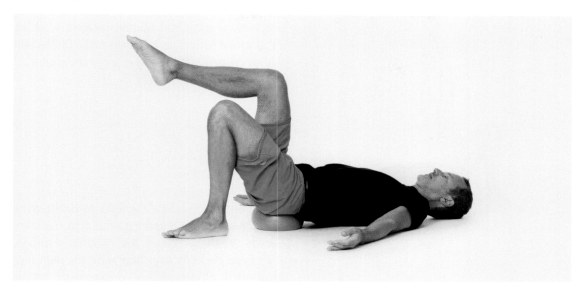

Variation: Lift both legs one after the other or simultaneously; in addition to the parallel position also incorporate internal and external rotations.

Effect of the ball: When doing the pelvic clock, the ball makes it easier to circle, increases motion awareness, and massages the sacrum. During the low abs exercise, it provides an unstable surface and makes it more difficult to stabilize the pelvis, improving abdominal strength and coordination.

IMPORTANT

Make sure the pelvis remains in a neutral position. Do not arch the back!

SINGLE-LEG CIRCLE

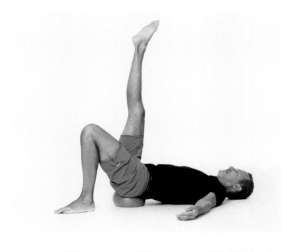

Starting position: On your back; the left knee is bent and the left foot is planted in extension of the sit bone; the right leg is extended to the ceiling and slightly rotated out; the ball is under the sacrum.

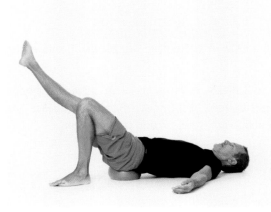

Execution: As you exhale, the right leg circles to the inside. As you inhale, the leg returns to the start. Repeat 5x, then circle in the opposite direction. Then bend the right knee and plant the right foot in extension of the sit bone. As you exhale, lift the left leg and as you inhale, extend it to the ceiling. Repeat everything with the left leg.

Variations: First stretch the supporting leg by pulling the bent playing leg into the chest with both hands, while simultaneously extending the supporting leg on the floor. Circle the leg to the inside, outside, and parallel to the hip.

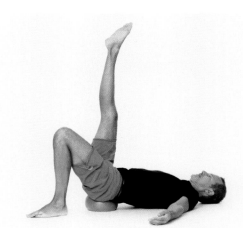

Effect of the ball: The ball increases the angle in the hip joint and makes it easier to extend the leg to the ceiling. It also requires more control during stabilization of the pelvis. When the supporting leg is extended on the floor, more hip extension is needed to keep the lumbar spine in a neutral position. Pulling the playing leg into the chest for the initial stretch while simultaneously extending the supporting leg provides a wonderful hip-flexor stretch.

IMPORTANT

Make sure the pelvis is in a neutral position. Do not arch the back!

ROLL UP

Starting position: Sit with your legs extended or knees bent and place the ball between your thighs or under the place in the spine where you have trouble rolling.

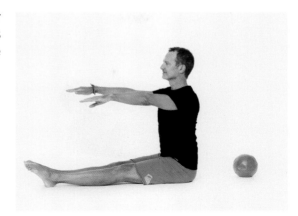

Execution: As you exhale, evenly roll the spine down. Once you are on your back or on the ball, inhale and then evenly roll back up as you exhale. Repeat 5-8x.

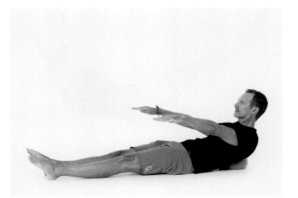

Effect of the ball: Holding the ball between the thighs helps to activate the adductors, the pelvic floor, and the deep abdominal muscles. Placing the ball under the spine allows you to work intensively in the area where you lack mobility or strength.

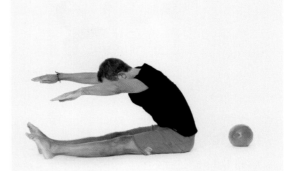

IMPORTANT

Roll vertebrae for vertebrae at an even pace. Keep your legs or feet firmly on the mat. Do not use momentum and don't bounce off the ball.

DOUBLE-LEG STRETCH

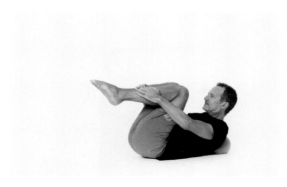

Starting position: On your back with the upper body lifted off the floor; legs are in a 90/90-degree position; hands rest on shins; the ball is held between the ankles or placed between the shoulder blades.

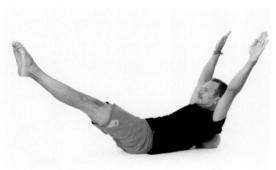

Execution: As you exhale, vigorously extend the legs forward while simultaneously extending the arms in the opposite direction. As you inhale, circle the arms to the outside towards your feet, bend the knees, and return to the starting position. Repeat 5-10x.

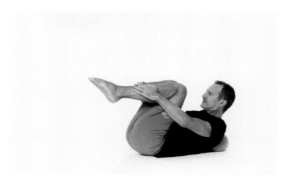

Effect of the ball: Holding the ball between your thighs helps to activate the adductors, the pelvic floor, and the deep abdominal muscles. Placing the ball between the shoulder blades helps maintain the position if the upper abdominals are weak and builds up the counteraction against the legs by pushing the sternum towards the ball.

IMPORTANT

Keep the pelvis and the lumbar spine in a neutral position. Lift the arms only as far towards the head as you are able to maintain shoulder alignment. Maintain balance between arm and leg extension. The ball between the shoulder blades is not a pillow!

SPINAL STRETCH

Starting position: Sit with your legs extended and more than shoulder-width apart. Hands rest on the ball in front of you between your legs; arms are extended. The ball is positioned under your hands.

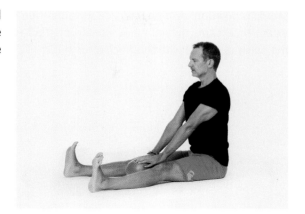

Execution: As you exhale, start to evenly roll forward leading with the head. As you do so, use firm pressure from your hands to roll the ball towards your feet. As you inhale, roll back up to an upright position. Repeat 3x.

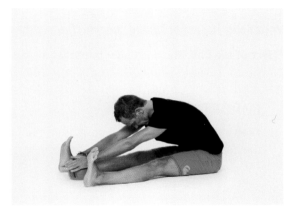

Effect of the ball: With pressure from the hands, the ball helps to activate the abdominal muscles and facilitates an even rolling motion. Use the ball to activate your core and create axial extension!

IMPORTANT

Keep the pelvis in a neutral position and firmly press the sit bones into the floor during the entire movement. Use your abdominal strength to roll the body down and up; don't just let it drop towards the floor.

DOUBLE-LEG LIFT

Starting position: In a neutral side-lying position with legs extended and closed. The head rests on the extended left arm; the right arm is bent with the hand resting in front of the chest. The ball is placed under the pelvis at a level with the Trochanter major.

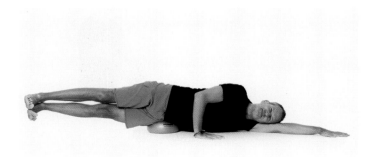

Execution: As you exhale, lift your closed legs off the floor. As you inhale, return them to the floor. Repeat 5x, then switch sides.

Variations: In case of limited shoulder flexion, the ball can also be placed under the head as a pillow.

Effect of the ball: The ball under the pelvis increases the range of motion and requires more balance.

IMPORTANT

Keep the pelvis in a neutral position in the frontal plane. To lift the legs, lengthen the side of the body resting on the floor; to lower the legs, lengthen the side of the body facing the ceiling.

SWAN DIVE

Starting position: Neutral supine position with legs closed; elbows are bent and hands are propped on the floor next to the ribcage; the ball is under the pelvis.

Execution: As you exhale, using your arms for support, roll the upper body up off the mat. As you inhale, extend the body into a long arch from the top of the head to the toes. As you exhale, let the upper body dive down as the legs swing upward like the rockers on a rocking horse. As you inhale, the upper body swings back up and the legs come down. Repeat 5-8x and then shake out the pelvis a bit.

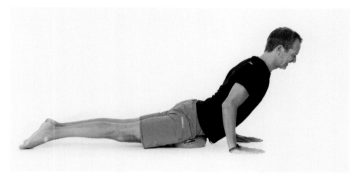

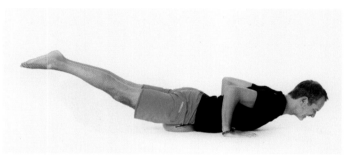

Effect of the ball: Placing the ball under the pelvis makes it easier to perform the rocking motion, improves awareness of a strong core, and helps participants with a lack of extension in the hips or thoracic spine. As an alternative, the ball can be held between the ankles. There it creates more axial length, improves engagement of adductors, pelvic floor, and deep abdominal muscles, and creates a more solid link between the core and the lower extremities.

IMPORTANT

Do not push your belly against the ball. Instead activate the body in depth, width, and length against the pressure of the ball.

DOUBLE-LEG KICK

Starting position: On your stomach in a neutral position with legs extended and closed; the head is turned to the right; the hands hold the ball in the hollow of the low back.

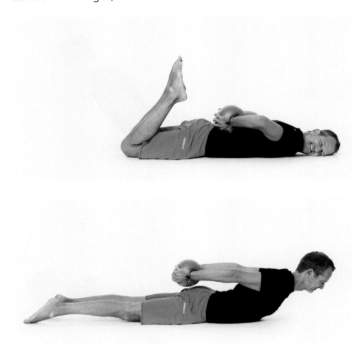

Execution: As you inhale, vigorously kick both heels towards the sit bones 2-3x. As you exhale, vigorously extend the legs on the floor. At the same time, squeeze the ball with your hands, extend the arms and lift the upper body, and turn the head to the other side. Then roll the upper body back down to the floor, release pressure on the ball, and move it back to the hollow of the low back. Still inhaling, kick the heels towards the sit bones again. Repeat 6-8x, then move into child's pose.

Effect of the ball: Squeezing the ball with the hands strengthens the arms, opens up the shoulders, activates the upper back, and creates axial length as well as extension of the thoracic spine.

IMPORTANT
The arms should be extended while squeezing the ball; otherwise work without the ball.

KNEE STRETCHES

Starting position: Neutral all-fours position with legs closed; the ball is placed under the shins near the kneecaps.

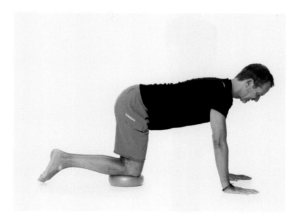

Execution: As you exhale, round the back from the crown of the head to the tailbone and pull the knees towards the hands. Breathe into the width of the back and return to the starting position. Roll the ball along the length of the shins. Repeat 5-8x, then move the back into extension and repeat the sequence.

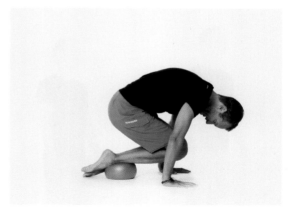

Variation: Start with a large ball under the feet and fully extend the legs back, and then bend them again to return to the starting position.

Effect of the ball: The ball under the shins facilitates the movement. Working with gentle pressure on the ball increases activation of the abdominal muscles.

IMPORTANT
Maintain trunk flexion or extension throughout the entire movement.

2 X 4

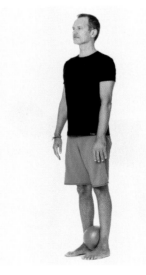

Starting position: Neutral standing position; the ball is held between the ankles.

Execution: Raise the heels off the floor, bend the knees, lower the heels back down to the floor, and vigorously extend the knees back into starting position. Repeat 3-4x, then reverse the movement sequence. Bend the knees, raise the heels, extend the knees, lower the heels, and return to the starting position. Repeat 3-4x.

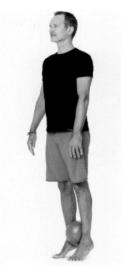
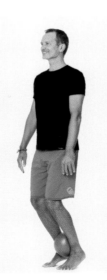
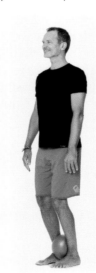
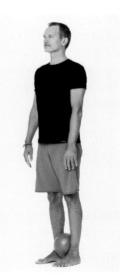

Effect of the ball: Holding the ball between the ankles improves the engagement of adductors, pelvic floor, and deep abdominal muscles, and creates a more solid connection between the core and the lower extremities. It helps to align legs and feet.

IMPORTANT
Keep the body as vertical as possible during the entire movement.

ALL OF THE EXERCISES AT A GLANCE

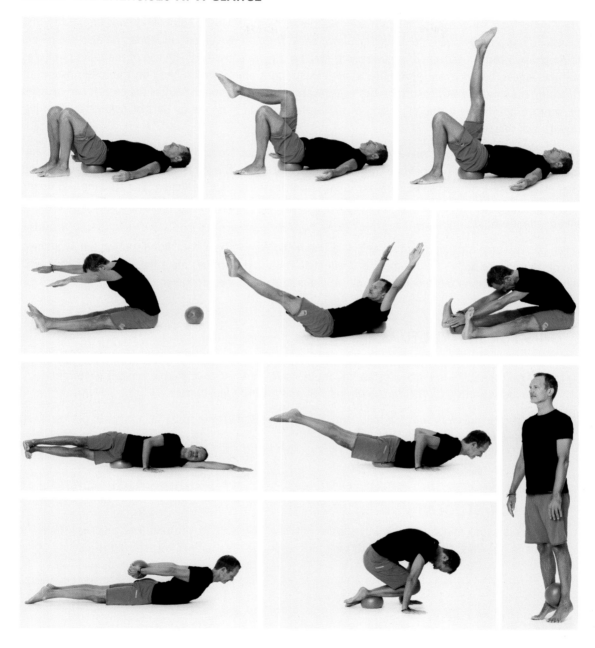

5.12.2 THE PILATES FOAM ROLLER

The Pilates foam roller originated with the Feldenkrais method. Moshe Feldenkrais was one of the first people to use a hardwood roller to improve awareness through movement. In Pilates we also use rollers to emphasize certain aspects of a movement, making it more conscious. The use of the roller promotes self-awareness, balance, and flexibility, as well as strength ability. When lying on the roller instead of the floor, the smaller contact surface improves awareness of the spine as well as the core. It can be used to improve nourishment and cleansing of tissue through self-massage as part of myofascial training (myofascial release).

The rollers increase the focus on centering and balance. The unstable position promotes intramuscular and intermuscular coordination, increases the use of muscles close to the joints, and promotes proprioception (self-awareness). Improved self-awareness greatly contributes to pain reduction. The student also learns that movement tasks can only be mastered by the entire body (functional units) instead of individual independently acting muscles.

It can be very successful in preventing as well as improving existing back pain. Blind spots in self-awareness are decreased, the body's nourishment is stimulated, the tissue becomes more flexible and resilient, and relaxing and loosening movement patterns are integrated via guided imagery.

TIPS FOR INSTRUCTORS

The roller should not be too firm and should not cause pain to the user. Place a mat, blanket, or towel over the roller to make it softer and more stable. Very sensitive people can get motion sick on the roller. Simply ask them to lie on the mat and they will feel better.

In the beginning, work with the roller only a few minutes at a time so participants can get used to the new challenge.

TIPS FOR STUDENTS

Roller massages should be felt but should not hurt. Be kind to yourself. The roller is often challenging. When you notice that it's too much, continue the exercises without the roller.

EXERCISE PROGRAM FOR THE PILATES FOAM ROLLER

BASIC BRIDGE

Starting position: With your back on the roller; knees are bent and feet are planted in extension of the sit bones; arms are extended alongside the roller, palms down.

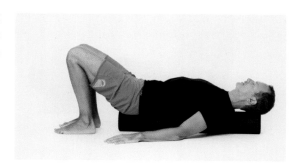

Execution: As you exhale, roll up evenly vertebrae by vertebrae, starting with the pelvis and up to the shoulder blades. With the next exhalation, roll down evenly, starting with the shoulder blades, back to starting position. Repeat 3-5x.

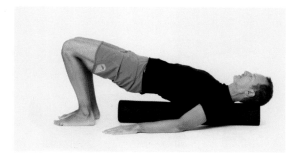

Easier: Plant the feet farther apart for more stability.

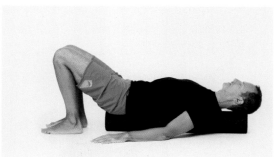

Effect of the ball: The roller improves awareness of the rolling motion. Having the feet lower than the pelvis makes it more challenging to lower the lumbar spine to the roller. The unstable surface requires more stability in hips and trunk.

IMPORTANT

If the roller's pressure on the spine is unpleasant, use a softer roller, place the mat on the roller for more comfort, or continue to practice without the roller.

LOW ABS, SINGLE-LEG STRETCH

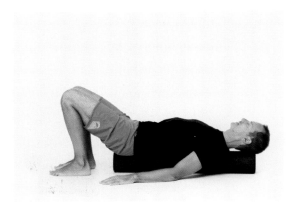

Starting position: With your back on the roller; knees are bent and feet are planted in extension of the spine; arms are extended alongside the roller, palms down.

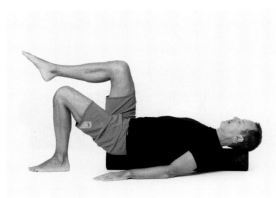

Execution: Alternately lift one leg off the mat and then lower it again. Lift the leg as you exhale and lower it as you inhale. Repeat 3-5x per leg.

Challenge: Let the arms float above the mat.

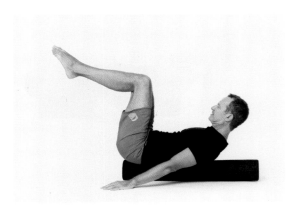

Then lift both legs as you exhale to move into tabletop position. The hands provide stability on the mat when you roll the upper body up with the next exhalation (sternum drop).

As you inhale, extend the right leg forward and move the left leg towards the chest. The pelvis remains neutral.

As you exhale, extend the left leg and bend the right leg towards the chest. Repeat 3-5x. Then extend the right as you exhale and bend the left, and then extend the left as you inhale and bend the right. Repeat 3-5x.

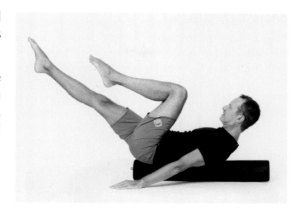

Effect of the roller: During the low abs exercise, the roller is an unstable surface that makes it more difficult to stabilize the pelvis and trunk. It improves abdominal strength and increases coordination. This effect is heightened during the single-leg stretch and the upper abdominals are activated considerably more.

IMPORTANT

Make sure the pelvis remains in a neutral position. Do not arch your back! Use your abdominal strength to lift the upper body and not the neck. Move your legs parallel during the single-leg stretch.

BASIC BRIDGING 2

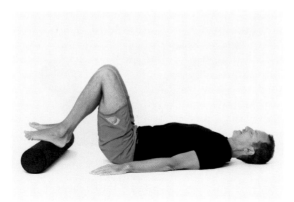

Starting position: On your back; knees are bent and feet are planted in extension of the sit bones; arms are extended alongside the body, palms down.

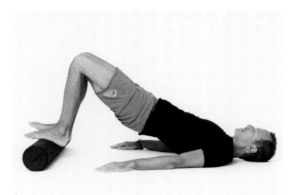

Execution: As you exhale, roll up evenly, vertebrae by vertebrae, starting with the pelvis and up to the shoulder blades. With the next exhalation, roll evenly from the shoulder blades back down to the starting position. Repeat 3-5x.

Challenge: On one leg.

Effect of the roller: The roller improves engagement of the hamstring muscles, promotes axial length, and requires more hip stability. The higher foot position makes rolling of the lumbar spine easier and allows the spine to roll up higher.

IMPORTANT

Vigorous hamstring activity can cause cramping in the back of the legs. Pressure from the roller against the soles of the feet can cause cramping in the feet. Roll up only as far as the shoulder girdle. Avoid excessive pressure on the head and neck.

MERMAID

Starting position: Z-seat with the right leg rotated out at the end of the roller and the right side of the pelvis resting on the roller; the left half of the pelvis floats next to the roller; the right hand is propped next to the pelvis on the roller for support and the left arm is extended to the ceiling.

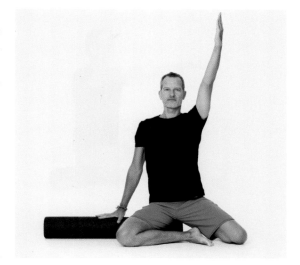

Execution: Inhale, let your left sit bone sink towards the floor, extend the left arm towards the ceiling, and lengthen your flank. As you exhale, bend to the right in a big arch, bend the right elbow, and allow the right shoulder to drop. As you inhale, return to the starting position. Repeat 3x. Then repeat the entire sequence on the other side.

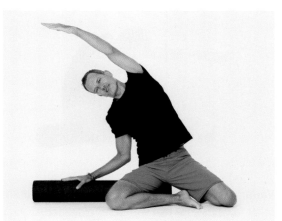

Effect of the roller: The roller compensates for a limited internal hip rotation and requires more balance.

IMPORTANT

Keep the pelvis neutral. Extend both flanks in a long arch and support yourself from the shortened side (do not cave in the side). As you move, imagine you are sandwiched between two panes of glass and you don't want to leave smudges on them.

SPINAL STRETCH

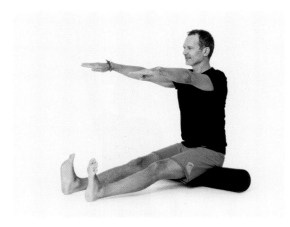

Starting position: Neutral seated position in the middle of the roller with legs extended and more than shoulder-width apart; arms are extended forward shoulder-width apart and parallel to the floor; palms face the floor.

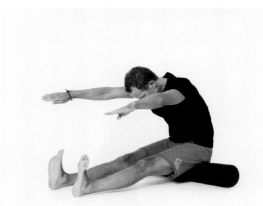

Execution: As you exhale, begin to roll forward evenly starting with the head. As you do so, extend the parallel arms forward towards the feet. As you inhale, roll back up to an upright seat. Repeat 3x.

Variations: Place the roller under the back of the knees. Place the roller on top of the shins and push the roller towards your feet with arms extended, using gentle pressure to support activation of the abdominal muscles.

Effect of the roller: The roller placed under the pelvis makes it easier for participants with tight muscles at the back of the legs to sit with their legs extended; it promotes the conscious pressing of the sit bones into the mat, and requires pelvic balance. When placed under the back of the knees, the roller makes it easier to sit. The roller placed under the hands helps to activate the abdominal muscles while rolling and supports an even rolling motion.

ADDUCTION, HIP MOBILIZATION

Starting position: Neutral side-lying position with the bottom leg extended on the mat and the top leg bent at 90/90-degree angles on top of the roller. The roller lies parallel to the practitioner in a vertical position; the bottom arm is extended below the head and the top arm is bent, the hand rests in front of the ribcage.

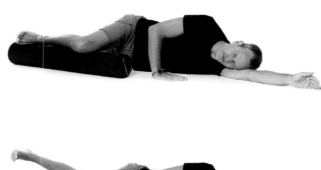

Execution: As you exhale, lift the extended bottom leg off the mat. Hold the foot in a flexed position and vigorously push out through the heel. As you inhale, return the leg to the mat. Repeat 5x.

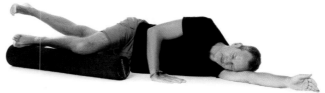

Next, place the bottom leg on the roller and roll the roller back and forth with the top leg. This mobilizes and maintains function of the hip joint and gently massages the adductors.

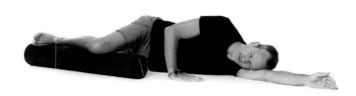

Switch sides and repeat the entire sequence.

Effect of the roller: The roller makes the movement easier during adduction by supporting the top leg, thereby facilitating pelvic stabilization.

IMPORTANT

Keep the pelvis in a neutral position in the frontal plane. To lift the bottom leg, actively lengthen it in the hip. Maintain a neutral lumbar spine while rolling.

SWAN DIVE

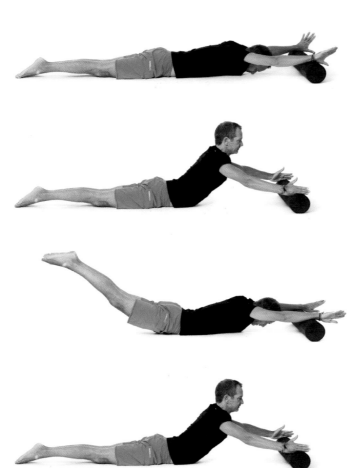

Starting position: Neutral prone position; arms are extended forward on the roller and at least shoulder-width apart with palms facing the floor; the roller is placed horizontally in front of the practitioner.

Execution: As you exhale, gently press the hands into the roller and use the shoulder blades to pull the roller towards the body and lift the trunk. As you inhale, return to the starting position. Repeat 3x.

Next, hold the trunk in the raised position and create a vigorous arch from the top of the head to the toes. As you exhale, roll the roller away from the body, lower the trunk, and lift the legs. As you inhale, roll the roller towards the body, lift the trunk, and lower the legs. Repeat 5-8x, then sit back in child's pose.

Effect of the roller: The roller supports shoulder mobility, promotes extension in the thoracic spine, helps maintain axial length, and keeps you centered during the movement.

IMPORTANT
In case of limited shoulder flexion, bend the elbows. Maintain axial length and a well-organized shoulder girdle.

STRETCHING DOG

Starting position: Neutral all-fours position with hands on the roller; roll alongside the mat.

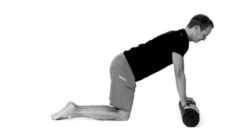

Execution: As you exhale, extend the right leg back parallel to the floor. Hold as you inhale. With the next exhalation, move the leg back to the starting position. Repeat with the left leg. Repeat 3x per leg.

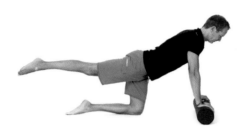

Next, place the roller under your shins in a horizontal position. Toes can touch the floor. As you exhale, extend the left arm and right leg parallel to the floor. Hold as you inhale, and as you exhale return to the starting position. Repeat on the other side. Repeat several times on each side.

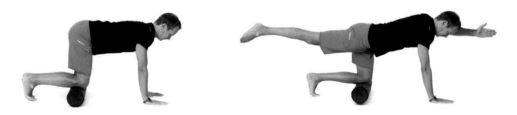

Effect of the roller: The roller promotes strength, coordination, and balance in the hips and shoulders.

IMPORTANT

Shoulder girdle and spine remain neutral. Keep this in mind as you lift the arm and leg. Work to create length and move the arm and leg from a stable trunk.

STANDING BALANCE

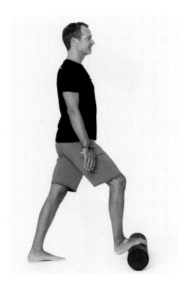

Starting position: Stand with one foot on top of the roller; the roller is placed horizontally in front of you on the floor.

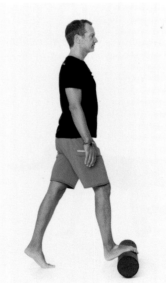
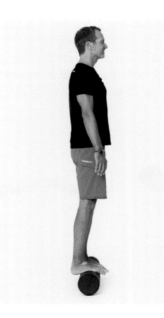

Execution: As you exhale, lift the heel of the foot that is on the floor, and lower it back down as you inhale. Repeat 3-5x, then switch sides.

Next, stand with both feet on the roller and balance there for several breaths (only for experienced practitioners; alternatively practice at a wall.)

Effect of the roller: Challenges the balancing ability.

IMPORTANT

When lifting the heel, place as little weight as possible on the roller. Keep the body as vertical as possible throughout the exercise.

ALL OF THE EXERCISES AT A GLANCE

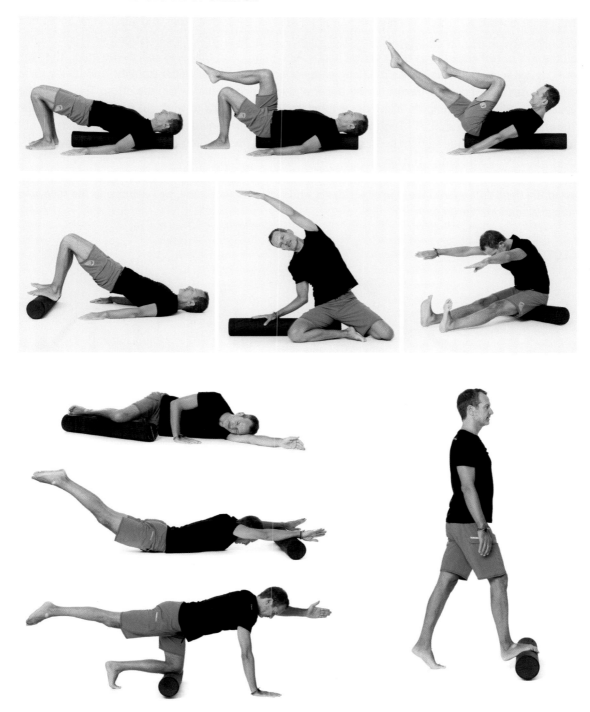

5.12.3 THE ELASTIC BAND

The elastic band is a classic among small props and extremely versatile. Arms and legs can be linked in a pseudo-closed chain. The possibilities are near endless, beginning with the easiest grip with both hands all the way to elaborate wraps that connect hands, feet, thighs, and calves, as well as the trunk. This type of body tension against resistance results in better alignment and thus more stability. And finally there are exercises that increase strength in the upper and lower extremities with little effort. The bands are available in different strengths, allowing even heterogeneous groups to work out together. But beware: The elastic bands pack a punch! People often underestimate how demanding the use of the bands is both for the instructor and the student because the idea is to work freestanding with the ability to move in any direction against resistance. The handling of the band as well as the combination of exercises should be well thought out beforehand. Otherwise the student is more focused on the wrap than the exercise. To avoid the band cutting into the skin or accidents while releasing the band, we recommend the following safe and comfortable wrap.

CLOTHESLINE WRAP

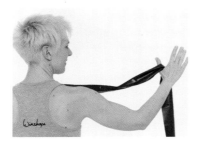 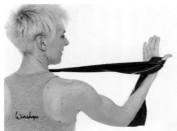 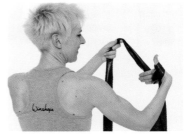

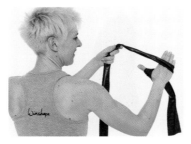 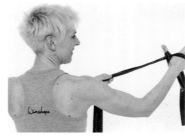

Place the short ends of the band between thumbs and forefingers in the direction of the pinkies. The tops of the hands point towards the user. Rotate the hands inward and lay the band across the tops of the hands and again between thumbs and forefingers.

TIPS FOR INSTRUCTORS

It is not necessary to structure an entire class around a small prop. Particularly in the beginning, it is enough to offer just 3-4 exercises, preferably with very few wrapping changes.

TIPS FOR STUDENTS

Use wraps that leave the hands open and avoid gripping the band or closing the hands. This has a positive effect on neck and shoulders.

PILATES

In this practice section we used the CLX-band by Theraband, though any type of resistance band will work. The continuous loops facilitate uncomplicated use and offer many more options than a traditional elastic band.

A medium-strength band approximately 2-2.5 m (6.5-8 feet) long is ideal for the exercises shown here.

FLOATING ARMS, ARM CIRCLE

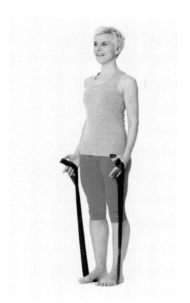

Starting position: Standing; stand on the band with both feet and hold the ends of the band in your hands.

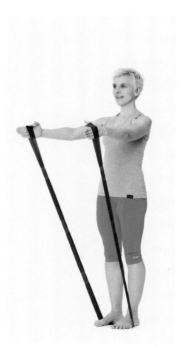
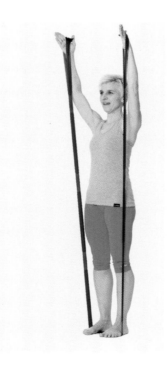

Execution: As you exhale, first let the shoulder blades drop and then extend the arms forward and up.

As you inhale, lower the arms back down. The shoulders stay down and the elbows are extended. Repeat 6-8x.

Variation: The same sequence to the sides and in circles.

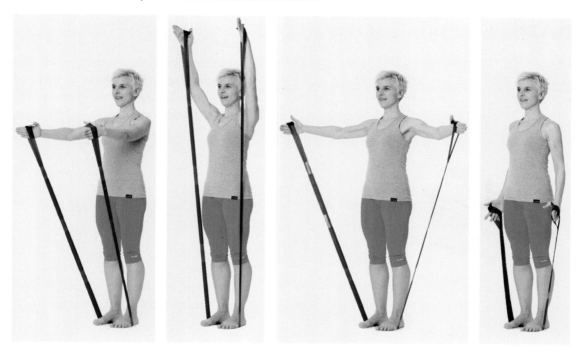

Effect of the band: The elastic band facilitates resistance training for more strength in the upper extremities. To do so, it links feet and hands, creating a pseudo-closed chain.

IMPORTANT

Watch the alignment of the shoulder girdle. Every arm movement begins with the hands pulling downward and shoulder blades dropping. The shoulders must be centered before the band's resistance can be felt.

EXERCISE PROGRAM WITH THE ELASTIC BAND

ROLL UP

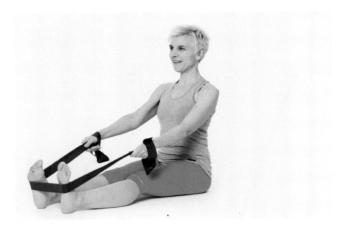

Starting position: Seated with legs extended forward; the band is stretched across the bottoms of the feet and the ends are held in the hands.

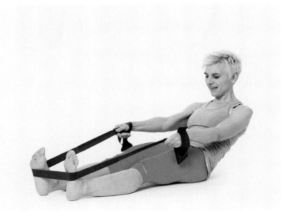

Execution: As you exhale, roll the spine down evenly starting at the pelvis.

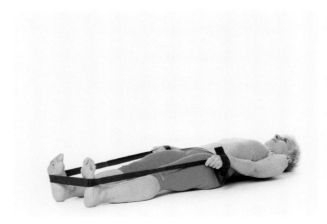

Inhale once you are down on your back, and then evenly roll back up with your next exhalation. Repeat 4-6x.

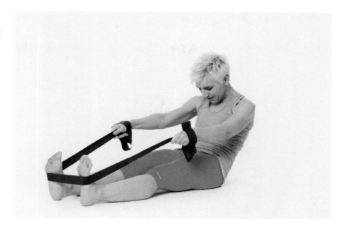

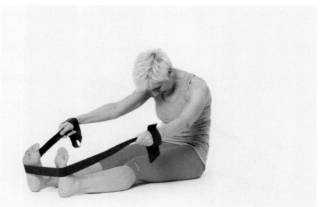

Effect of the elastic band: The elastic band makes it easier to roll down incrementally.

IMPORTANT

The arms remain extended. The idea is to work against the resistance while rolling down and up again. The band is not used to pull up.

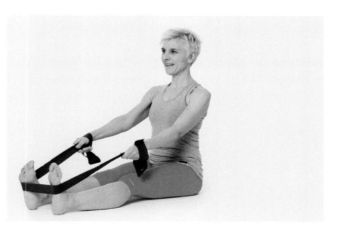

DOUBLE-LEG STRETCH

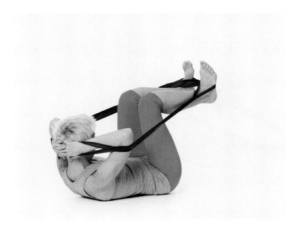

Starting position: On your back with legs in a 90/90-degree position; the band is stretched across the soles of both feet, the ends are held in the hands; arms are crossed behind the head.

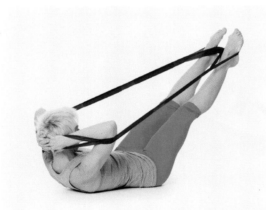

Execution: As you exhale, extend both legs forward at a slant, and as you inhale, return to the starting position.

Repeat 6-8x.

Effect of the elastic band: Connecting the lower and upper body makes it easier to control the leg movement. The band partially supports the weight of the legs.

SINGLE-LEG CIRCLE

Starting position: On your back; the band is stretched across the sole of the left foot and both ends are held in the left hand. The left leg is extended to the ceiling for a stretch and slightly externally rotated in the hip; the right arm is extended to the side on the floor.

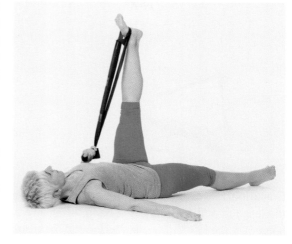

Execution: As you exhale, circle the left leg to the outside and as you inhale move it across the body back to the starting position. The semi-circle to the outside can be dynamic and sweeping.

Repeat 4-6x per side.

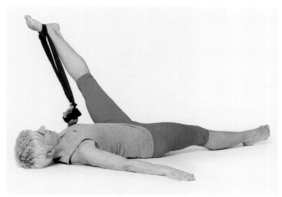

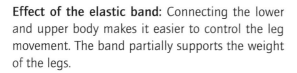

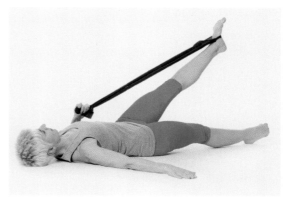

Effect of the elastic band: Connecting the lower and upper body makes it easier to control the leg movement. The band partially supports the weight of the legs.

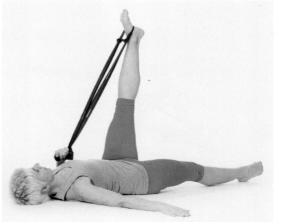

TIP

Some participants find holding the band in the opposite hand more comfortable.

SAW

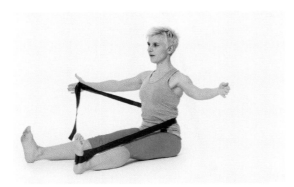

Starting position: Seated with legs extended shoulder-width apart; arms are laterally extended at shoulder-level; the band is looped around the sole of the left foot, across the back, and held in the right hand; there is continuous tension on the band.

Execution: As you inhale, turn the trunk to the right and relax the band. As you exhale, turn the trunk to the left and add tension to the band. After several repetitions, add a forward bend and move the right hand past the left foot while tracking the backward movement of the left hand.

Repeat each version 4-6x per side.

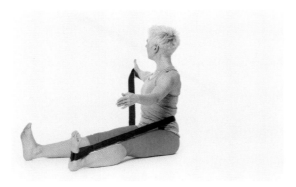

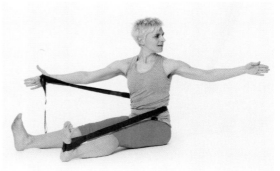

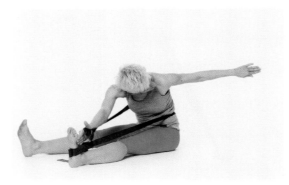

Effect of the elastic band: Execution with and without resistance. The movement results in more body tension and thus in greater range of motion.

IMPORTANT
The pelvis remains steady.

STRETCHING DOG

Starting position: On all fours; the band is anchored around the left foot and under both hands.

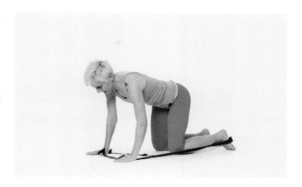

Execution: As you exhale, extend the left leg back and as you inhale, bend it again. At the same time, the right arm extends forward. As you inhale, return to the starting position.

Repeat 4-6x per side.

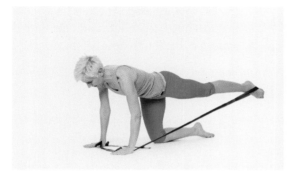
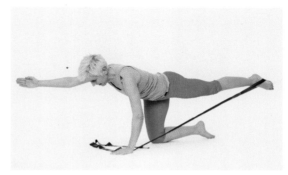

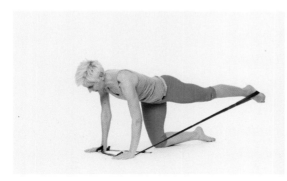
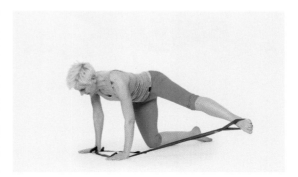

Variation: Extend the right leg back, then rotate it out and move it to the side and back again; arms remain on the floor.

Effect of the elastic band: Connecting the lower and upper body makes it easier to control the leg movement.

SIDE KICK

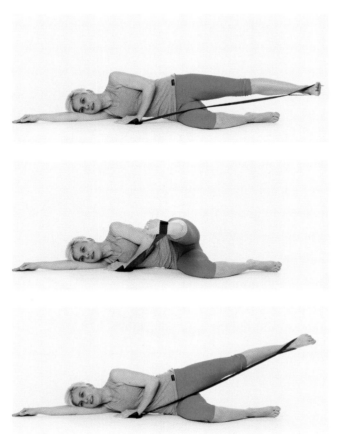

Starting position: Lie on your right side with the right bottom leg bent and the left top leg extended in extension of the spine; the band is looped around the left foot and the ends are held under the left hand; the left hand is propped on the floor in front of the chest and secures the band to the floor.

Execution: As you inhale, flex the left hip and move the extended left leg forward; the left foot is flexed. As you exhale, move the extended leg back until the hip is extended; the foot is now pointed.

Repeat 4-6x per side.

Variation: Do the exercise in a forearm side plank with the pelvis lifted.

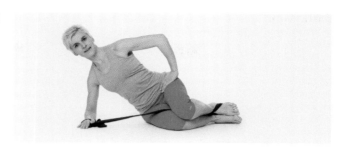

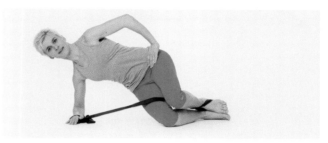

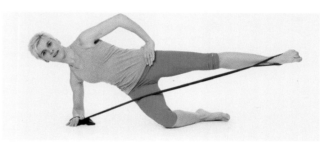

Effect of the elastic band: The execution of the movement with and against resistance creates more body tension and thus results in greater range of motion.

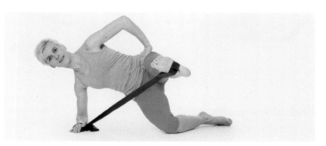

IMPORTANT

Participants should first be able to execute the Pilates exercise side kick with technical accuracy. Execution with the elastic band is more challenging with respect to alignment because more elements must be coordinated.

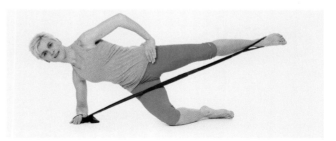

SWIMMER

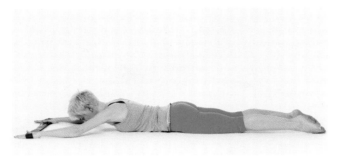

Starting position: On your stomach; the band is folded in half and held with both hands, adding tension.

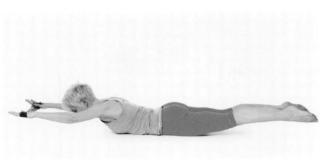

Execution: Gently extend the entire body so the upper body and legs are raised off the floor. Now paddle arms and legs on a diagonal while maintaining tension on the band and breathe evenly. Paddle five times for each inhalation and five times for each exhalation. Breathe evenly.

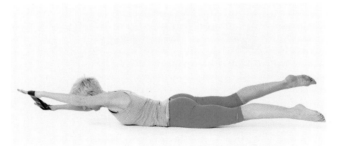

Effect of the elastic band: Using the outside of the pinkies to stretch the elastic band creates better alignment in the shoulder girdle.

IMPORTANT
You must stay centered during the paddling movements!

ALL OF THE EXERCISES AT A GLANCE

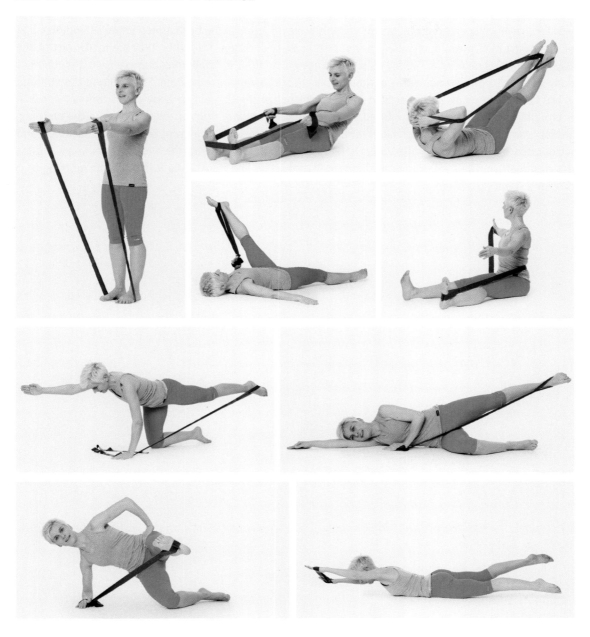

5.13   GOOD MORNING!

Have you ever watched small children or animals wake up after having been asleep for an extended period of time? First they yawn loudly, then they stretch in every direction. After that, they are ready to start the day. Our muscles relax when we are asleep and need a stimulus to build up enough tension again for our daily activities. Yawning generates oxygen uptake to stimulate our circulation. Stretching in the morning is like taking the wrinkles that settled in overnight out of the tissue. Our bodysuit of connective tissue is brought back into shape and refitted. A good exercise program right after getting up in the morning, chases away fatigue, clears the head, and stimulates fat oxidation. It simply makes us feel well and invigorated. You can get a similar effect after a long trip in the car or at the end of a seemingly endless day at the office. The exercise progression targets activation and is just as refreshing in the morning as it is after a strenuous meeting.

TIP FOR INSTRUCTORS

Only use this series if your participants can be active after the class. It is not suitable as a workout in the evening. We have a "Good Night" program for that.

TIP FOR STUDENTS

This series helps your day get off to a good start, particularly during the dark time of the year.

THE GOOD MORNING EXERCISE PROGRAM

WAKE UP

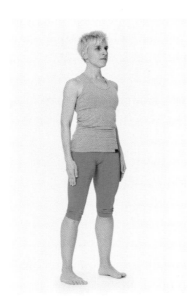

Starting position: Standing; feet are shoulder-width apart.

Execution: As you inhale, extend the arms to the ceiling; the sternum pulls diagonally forward and up. Build up tension in the front of the body and stay centered. As you exhale, circle the arms back and up until they are extended forward, and simultaneously do a squat.

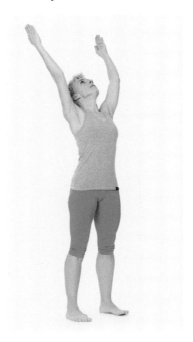 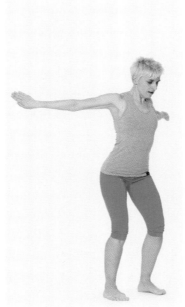 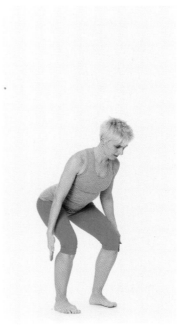

As you inhale, lower the arms to the floor, leading with the outside of the pinkies to stretch the back; the sit bones push back and up. As you exhale, relax and roll the spine up again. Repeat 4-6x.

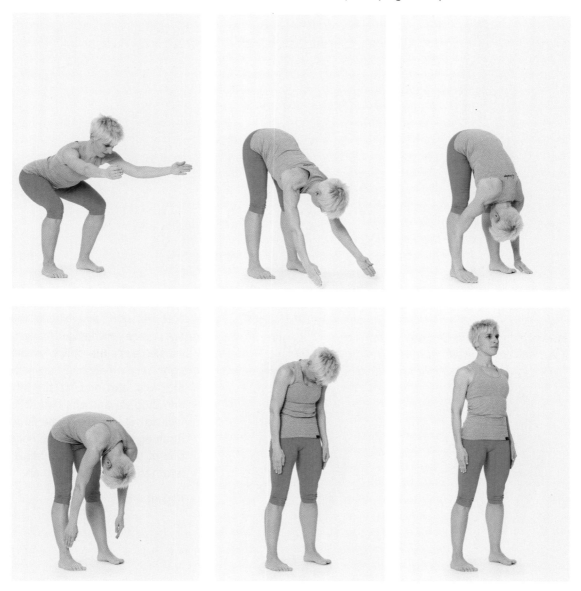

TIP

In the beginning, keep the knees bent as you roll up. After 3-4 repetitions you can change the progression as shown in the photos.

SIDE BEND, STANDING

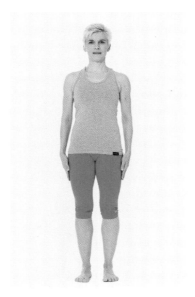

Starting position: Standing; feet are hip-width apart.

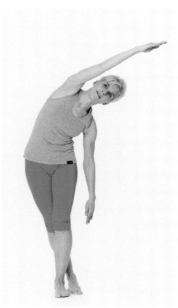
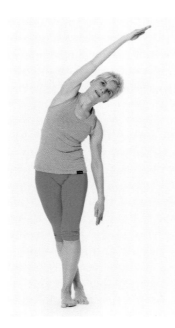

Execution: Cross the left leg over the right and extend the right arm overhead. As you exhale, push the pelvis to the right, reach diagonally up with the right arm and let the left arm drop towards the floor. The feet actively press into the floor, resulting in a stretch of the right side of the body. As you inhale, return to the starting position.

Repeat 6-8x.

TIP
Add small pulses at the end of the stretch.

STANDING SAW

Starting position: Standing straddle.

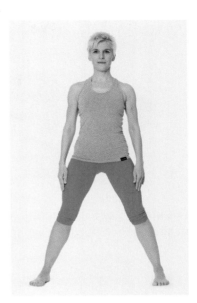

Execution: As you inhale, extend the arms to the sides. As you exhale, shift your weight to the left leg and bend the left knee. As you exhale, reach for the left foot with your right hand; the spine rotates and your glance moves past the right hand and into space. The iliac crests are level and parallel to the floor. As you inhale, return to an upright position.

Repeat 6-8x.

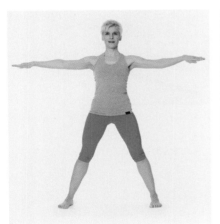 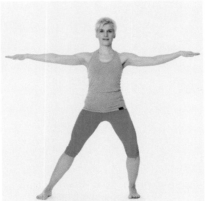 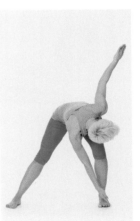

Variation: Rotate the legs out slightly.

TIP
Rotation increases as the hand continues to reach further towards the outside of the foot.

⚡ PILATES

ONE HUNDRED

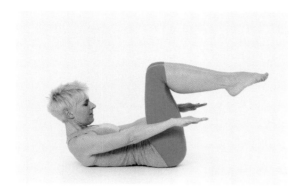

Starting position: On your back; legs are in tabletop position; head and shoulder girdle are rolled up (sternum drop); arms are extended alongside the body, palms down.

Execution: Take 5 quick breaths and then exhale quickly 5x while vigorously pumping the arms using a small range of motion. Repeat up to 10x.

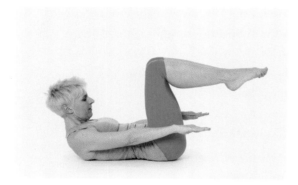 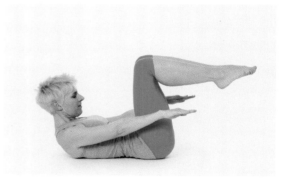

TIP
Incrementally build up your breathing: first inhale 2x and exhale 2x, 3x, 4x, etc.

ROLLING BACK

Starting position: Seated balance; hands rest on knees.

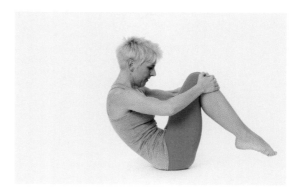

Execution: As you inhale, shift your weight back and roll backwards up to the shoulder girdle. As you exhale, roll back up into a seated balance. Repeat 6-8x.

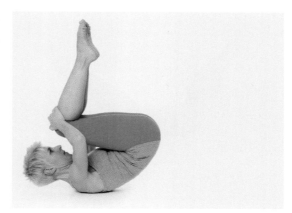

TIP
Maintain the spine's rounded C-shape throughout the exercise. The movement always begins and ends in a balance.

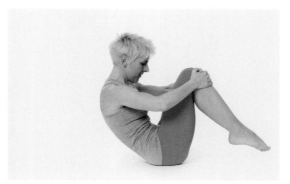

DOUBLE-LEG STRETCH

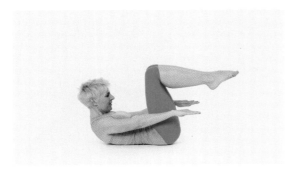

Starting position: On your back; sternum drop; knees in towards the body.

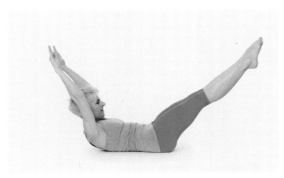

Execution: As you exhale, extend the arms and legs; as you inhale, return to the starting position.

Repeat 4-6x per side.

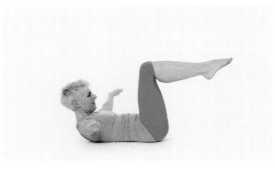

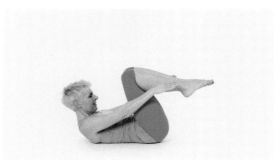

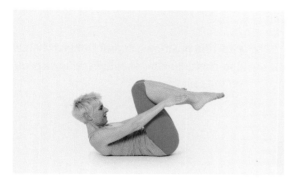

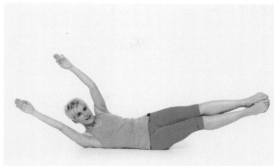

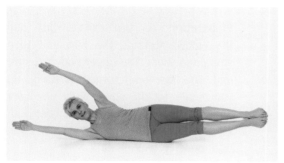

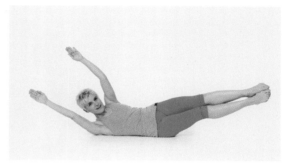

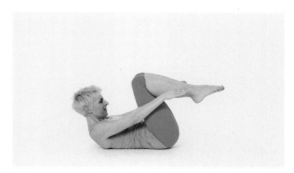

Variation: As you open up the body, turn over onto your side, then turn back over onto your back.

Repeat 4x per side.

SWAN DIVE

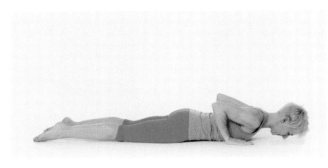

Starting position: On your stomach; hands are planted below shoulders; elbows point to the ceiling.

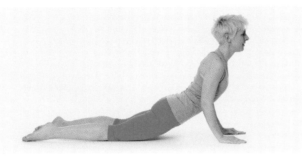

Preparation: As you exhale, first pull the elbows towards the feet and then straighten them. The upper body extends, and the sternum pushes forward. As you inhale, let the upper body sink back down. With the next exhalation, raise both extended legs off the floor, and lower them back down as you inhale.

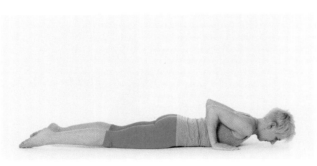

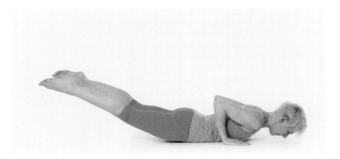

Starting position: On your stomach; hands are planted below shoulders; elbows are extended.

As you exhale, release the hands and roll forward along the front of the body up to the sternum. Legs are fully extended and raised. As you inhale, rock back and plant your hands back on the floor.

Repeat 4-6x.

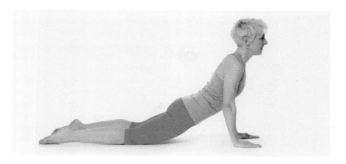

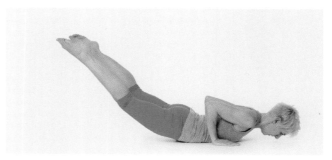

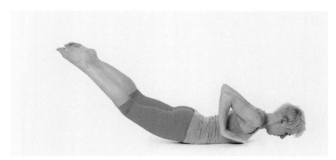

IMPORTANT

Stay centered and maintain axial length. At the end of the exercise, move into child's pose for several breaths to relax the back.

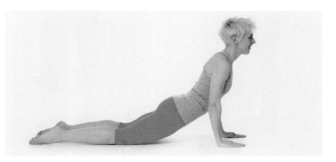

PUSH-UP

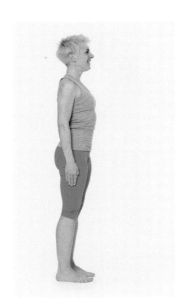

Starting position: Standing; feet are hip-width apart.

Execution: As you exhale, roll the spine down, as you inhale, walk your hands forward into plank.

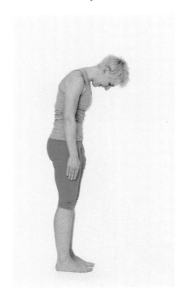 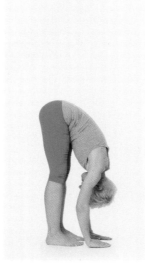 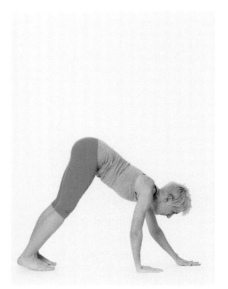

As you exhale, extend into the up stretch; as you inhale, walk your hands to your feet; as you exhale, roll up to standing.

Repeat 4 x.

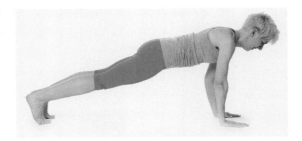

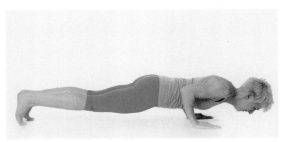

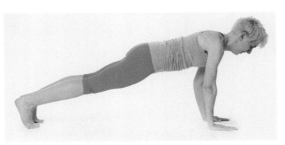

TIP
These exercises can be combined into a series by adding one new element to each repetition.

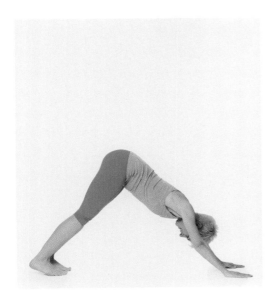

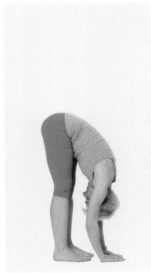

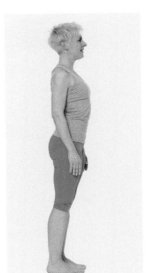

PILATES

ALL OF THE EXERCISES AT A GLANCE

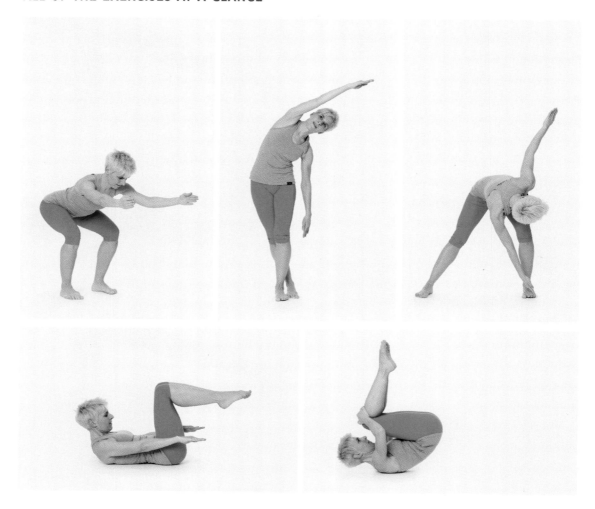

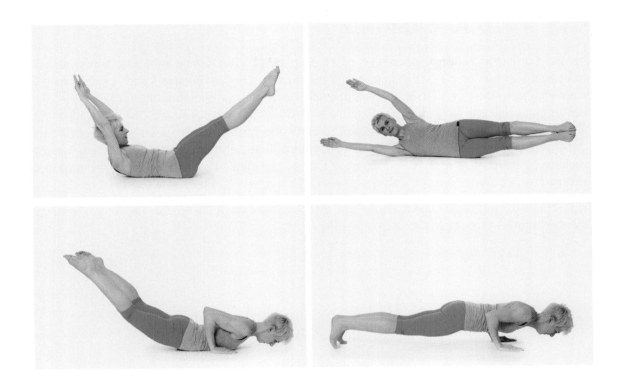

5.14   GOOD EVENING!

Evening is a time of rest and regeneration, of refueling and building. Gentle movement combined with slow breaths as well as loosening stretches are helpful here. Gentle movements and stretches release tension resulting from extended sitting, one-sided movements, and overloading during our daily lives. Calm breaths that emphasize exhalation stimulate the parasympathetic nervous system. The parasympathetic nervous system is responsible for processes of recovery and synthesizing processes in the body. These cannot take place in situations of physical or mental stress. That is also why a tough, demanding workout would be counterproductive during this phase of the day. You should also avoid deep backbends as they wake you up and energize you. Instead choose gentle forward bends as they allow you to let go.

This program consists of gentle exercises for your regeneration. It clears the head and allows you to let go. And dinner tastes even better after a little exercise.

TIPS FOR INSTRUCTORS

This exercise program will allow your participants to power down and unwind. If you wish to wake your participants up and get them moving, you should choose a different exercise sequence like, for instance, our "Good Morning" exercise program.

TIPS FOR STUDENTS

Even when you feel like just lying on the couch, after this exercise program you will be much better able to leave the day behind. And it only takes 15 minutes!

♙ PILATES

EXERCISE PROGRAM FOR THE EVENING

BREATHING, PELVIC TILT, BRIDGING

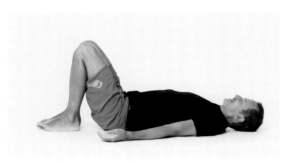

Starting position: On your back with knees bent and feet planted; arms rest alongside the body; palms face the ceiling.

Execution: Begin by taking long, slow breaths. Emphasize exhalation. Relax the abdominal wall as you exhale and activate the ribs and thoracic spine by breathing deeply and broadly into the ribcage. Take several breaths until your breaths flow calmly and evenly.

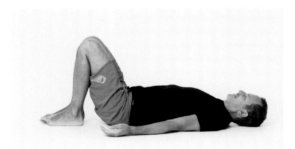 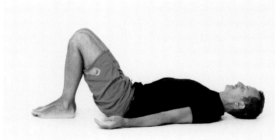

Now gently tilt the pelvis in time with the breath to loosen up the low back and hips. As you exhale, roll towards the lumbar spine; as you inhale, roll towards the tailbone. Repeat several times.

As you exhale, evenly roll the entire spine up off the mat starting with the pelvis and no farther than the shoulder blades. Consciously extend your hips without creating tension in the low back. With your next exhalation, starting at the sternum, roll back down to the starting position. Imagine your warm breath is melting the front of your body. Repeat 3-4x.

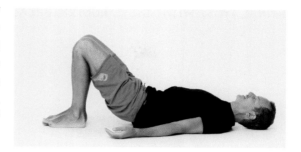

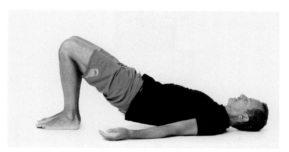

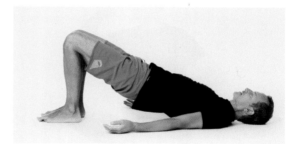

Variation: Extend one leg on the floor and roll up into bridge. Let the pelvis turn towards the side with the extended leg and gently rotate the spine.

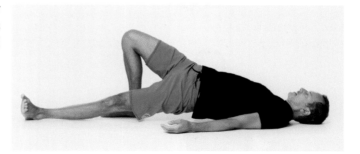

TIP

To relax the neck, you can place a towel or a pillow under your head while taking the breaths and doing the pelvic tilts. But please remove it before doing the bridging to protect the neck.

SPINAL TWIST WITH SINGLE-NOSTRIL BREATHING

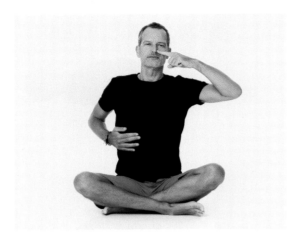

Starting position: Neutral seated position with legs crossed.

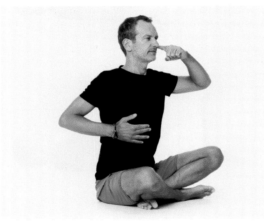

Execution: Rest the right hand against the right side of the ribcage and seal your left nostril with your left hand. As you inhale, breathe into the right half of the ribcage and twist to the right. Repeat three times, and then repeat everything on the left side.

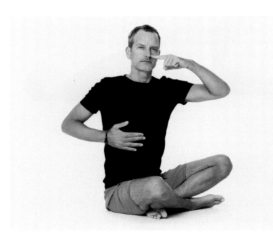

TIP

Breathe slowly and evenly. Inhaling during rotation creates more space between the ribs. You can also practice alternate-nostril breathing without the twist. It harmonizes the respiratory flow of the left and right nostril and balances their energies.

BOOK OPENING, RIGHT

Starting position: In a side-lying position; legs are in a 90/90-degree position; the head is supported; the arms are extended and stacked in front of the tip of the sternum.

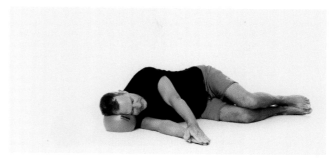

Execution: As you inhale, slide the left arm forward on top of the right arm. As you exhale, release the left arm and start to roll over onto your back. Track the left hand with your eyes. When the spinal rotation is complete, take a breath and extend both arms towards the walls, then return to the starting position as you exhale. Repeat 2-3x.

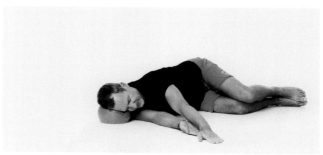

Variation: Only slide the top arm forward and back to activate the shoulder and shoulder blade.

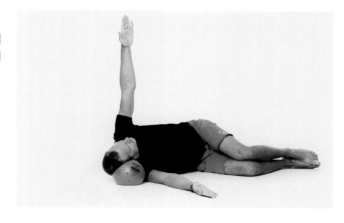

TIP
Consciously press the bottom arm into the mat and lengthen it through the fingertips to create more space between the shoulder blades and increase rotation.

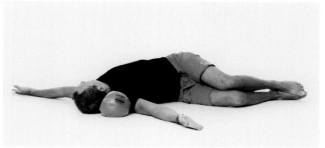

SUPINE SIDE BEND

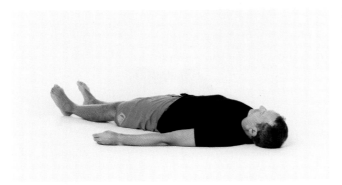

Starting position: On your back with legs extended and hip-width apart; arms are extended alongside the body; palms face the ceiling.

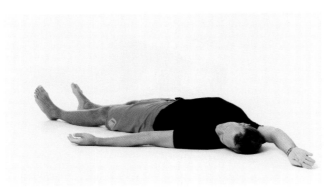

Execution: As you exhale, slide the right arm to the side and up overhead on the floor while bending to the left. Next cross the right leg over the left leg and make it really long. You will look like a banana from above. Hold this position for several breaths and return to the starting position. Repeat 1-2x per side.

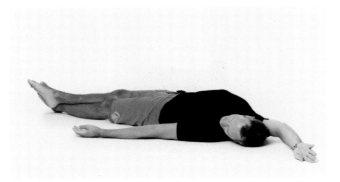

TIP
The motion is more like a languorous stretch. Yawn if you feel like it.

BOOK OPENING, LEFT

Starting position: Side-lying position; legs are in a 90/90-degree position; the head is supported; arms are stacked and extended forward in front of the tip of the sternum.

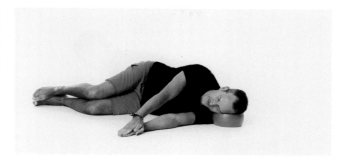

Execution: As you inhale, slide the left arm forward on top of the right arm. As you exhale, release the left arm and start rolling over onto your back. Track the left hand with your eyes. When the spinal rotation is complete, take a breath and extend both arms towards the walls. Return to the starting position as you exhale. Repeat 2-3x.

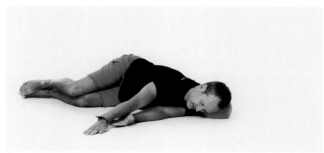

Variation: Only slide the top arm forward and back to activate the shoulder and shoulder blade.

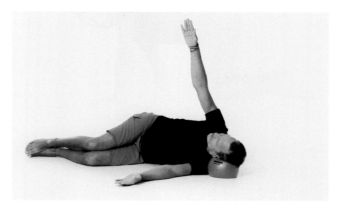

TIP
Consciously press the bottom arm into the mat and lengthen it through the fingertips to create more space between the shoulder blades and increase rotation.

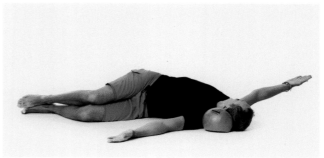

THREAD THE NEEDLE

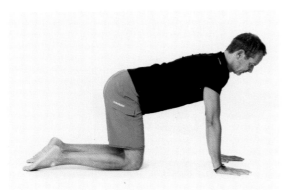

Starting position: Neutral all-fours position.

Execution: As you exhale, slide the left hand under your right arm with the palm facing the ceiling. As you do so, bend the right elbow for a clean rotation. As you inhale, return to the starting position. Repeat 3x, then switch sides.

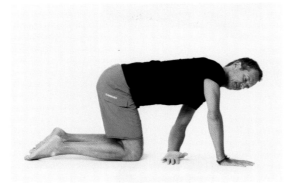 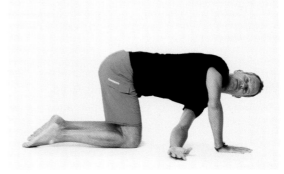

TIP

Start the movement with your eyes and move them in the direction of the desired rotation. Pull the sit bones back for axial length and stability.

SPINAL STRETCH

Starting position: Sit with your legs extended forward and about mat-width apart; arms rest on the floor next to the legs; palms face the ceiling.

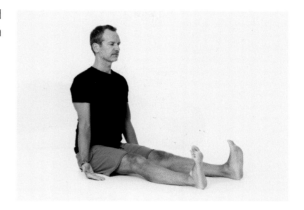

Execution: As you exhale, roll forward vertebrae by vertebrae starting with the head. As you do so, let the hands slide forward alongside the legs. Elbows remain slightly bent. Hold the forward bend for two breaths, then roll back up to an upright seated position as you inhale. Repeat up to 3x.

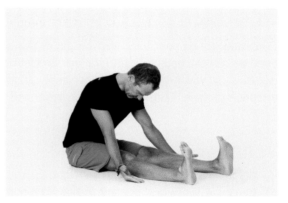

TIP

Imagine sitting against a wall—or actually sit against a wall—and roll up and down against the wall. If necessary, bend the knees or use a raised seat. Look in the direction of movement. To relax, place a bolster or large pillow on your thighs to rest your upper body on.

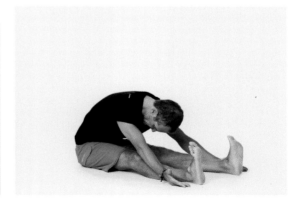

BREATHING

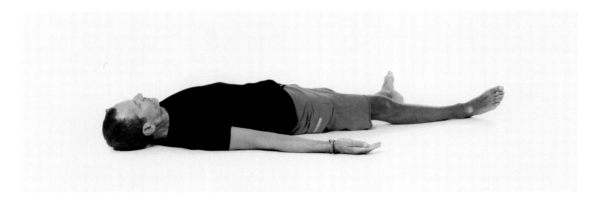

Starting position: On your back with legs extended or knees bent; arms rest alongside the body; palms face the ceiling.

Execution: Lie on your back like you did at the beginning of this exercise program, and reflect on the exercises. Let the body melt into the mat and let go. If you can still feel tension in your body, consciously release it as you exhale. Afterwards simply allow your thoughts to flow through you without paying attention to them. Relax your body and your mind.

TIP

It's impossible not to think. Therefore, accept your thoughts yet do not turn them over in your mind, but simply let them go. With a little practice, your mind will become calmer and not jump from thought to thought like a curious monkey.

ALL OF THE EXERCISES AT A GLANCE

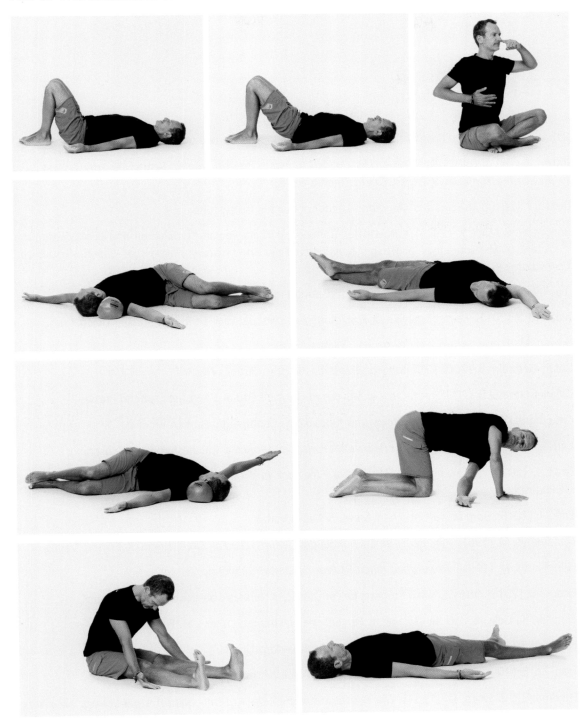

APPENDIX

REFERENCES

Barral, J. P. (2013). *Die Botschaften unseres Körpers.* München: Südwest Verlag.

Barth, C. A. (2005). *Das neue Denkmodell in der Physiotherapie: Bewegungsentwicklung und Bewegungskontrolle.* Stuttgart: Georg Thieme Verlag.

Beach, P. (2010). *Muscles and Meridians.* London: Churchill Livingstone.

Benzer, W. & Mayr, K. (2013). Körperliches Training zur Therapie von Krankheiten und Beschwerden des Alters. In M. Wonisch et. al (Hrsg.), *Kompendium der Sportmedizin: Physiologie, Innere Medizin und Pädiatrie* (S. 457-462). Berlin: Springer.

Black, M. (2015). *Centered.* Pencaitland: Handspring Publishing Ltd.

Blom, M. J. (2012). *Pilates and Fascia, Fascia: the tensional network.* London: Churchill Livingston.

Bowen, M. Internetseite. Historie von J. H. Pilates

Calais-Germain, B. (2005). *Anatomy of Breathing.* Seattle: Editions Des Iris.

Calais-Germain, B. (2007). *Anatomy of Movement* (Revised Edition). Seattle: Eastland Press.

Clippinger, K. (2007). *Dance anatomy and Kinesiology.* Champaign: Human Kinetics.

Earls, J. & Myers, T. (2010). *Fascial Release for Functional Balance.* Chichester: Lotus Publishing.

Earls, J. (2014). *Born to walk – Myofascial Efficiency and the body in movement.* Chichester: Lotus Publishing.

Earls, J. (2016). *Born to walk.* Aachen: Meyer & Meyer Verlag.

Feldenkrais, M. (1981). *Abenteuer im Dschungel des Gehirns: Der Fall Doris.* Berlin: Suhrkamp Verlag.

Feldenkrais, M. (1996). *Bewußtheit durch Bewegung.* Berlin: Suhrkamp Verlag.

Fitogram, (2016), https://www.fitogram.de/pro/articles/pilates-websites-analyse-und-tipps

Fletcher, R., Liekens, B. & San Miguel, L. Persönliche Erzählungen über J. H. Pilates.

Franklin, E. (1999). *Befreite Körper.* Kirchzarten: VAK Verlags GmbH.

Franklin, E. (2000). *Entspannte Schultern, gelöster Nacken.* München: Kösel Verlag.

Friedman, P. & Eisen, G. (1984). *The Pilates Method of Physical and Mental Conditioning.* New York: Warner Books.

Friedman, P. & Eisen, G. (2004). *The Pilates Method of Physical and Mental Conditioning.* New York: Viking Studio.

Gallagher, S. & Kryzanowska, R. (1999). *The Pilates Method of Body Conditioning.* Philadelphia (PA): BainBridgeBooks.

Geweniger, V. & Bohlander, A., (2012). *Das Pilates-Lehrbuch.* Berlin Heidelberg: Springer-Verlag GmbH.

Guimberteau, J. C. (2004). *Strolling under the Skin.* Paris: Elsevier.

Historische Pilates Videos von M. Bowen und Power Pilates

Ingber, D. (1998). The Architecture of Life. *Scientific American January*, 48-57.

Laarz, D. (2017) Atem. *Geo Magazin, (02)* 42-50

Langevin, H. (2006). Connective Tissue: a bodywide signaling network? *Medical Hypotheses, 66* (6), 1074-1077.

Larkam E., verschiedene Ausbildungsskripte und Videos

Lederman, E. (2013). *Therapeutic Stretching: toward a functional approach.* Edinburgh: Churchill Livingston.

Lee, D. (2011) *The Pelvic Girdle: An Integration of clinical expertise and research* (4. Aufl.) Edinburgh: Elsevier.

Lessen, D. (2013). *The PMA Pilates Certification Exam Study Guide.* 3. Aufl. Miami: PMA Inc.

Lexy, H. (2011). Dissertation – *Eine explorative Querschnittsstudie zur Darstellung der Interaktion zwischen Muskeln und Knochen bei Senioren-Master-Athleten während der 15. Leichtathletik-Europameisterschaften.* Berlin: Charité – Universitätsmedizin

McDougall, C. (2010). *Born to run.* München: Karl Blessing Verlag.

Müller, D. & Hertzer, K. (2015). *Training für die Faszien.* München: Südwest Verlag.

Myers, T. (2001). *Anatomy Trains.* Edinburgh: Churchill Livingston.

Opitz, S., (2013). *Pilates als bewegungstherapeutische Methode bei Depressionen.* Hamburg: Dr. Kovac.

Pilates, J. H. (1934). *Your Health.* Nachdruck 1998. Presentation Dynamics Inc.

Pilates, J. H. & Miller, W. R. (1945). *Return to Life through Contrology.* Nachdruck 2003. Presentation Dynamics Inc.

Pilates Bodymotion. *Ausbildungsskripte*

Richardson, C., Hodges, P. & Hides, J. (2009) *Segmentale Stabilisation im LWS- und Beckenbereich* (1. Aufl.) München: Urban & Fischer.

Richter, P. & Hebgen, E. (2011). *Triggerpunkte und Muskelfunktionsketten.* Stuttgart: Haug Verlag.

Rincke, E. (2015). *Joseph Pilates: Der Mann dessen Name Programm wurde.* Freiburg im Breisgau: Verlag Herder.

Rolf, I.P. (1977) *Rolfing: The integration of Human Structures.* New York: Fitzhenry & Whiteside Ltd.

Schleip, R. & Müller, D. (2012). Training Principles for fascial connective tissue – Scientific Foundation and suggested applications. *Journal of Bodywork and Movement Therapy, 1-13.*

Schleip, R. (2011). *Principles of Fascia Fitness.* www.terra-rosa.com. Issue 7

Schleip, R. & Bayer, J. (2014). *Faszien Fitness.* München: Riva.

Starrett, K. & Murphy, T. J. (2015). *Ready to run.* München: Riva.

Tittel, K. (2003). *Beschreibende und funktionelle Anatomie des Menschen* (14. Aufl.) Amsterdam: Elsevier Urban & Fischer.

Vleeming, A., Mooney, V. & Stoeckart, R. (2007). *Movement, Stability and Lumbarpelvic pain* (2. Aufl.) Churchill, Livingston, Elsevier.

Vleeming, A. et al. (2014). The coupling of paraspinal muscles. *Journal of Anatomy.*

http://www.pflaum.de/pt/archiv/a_pt_16_01_p06.pdf

https://de.wikipedia.org/wiki/Hypermobilit%C3%A4tssyndrom

CREDITS

Cover and interior design:	Sannah Inderelst, Annika Naas
Layout:	Bruno Hilger, www.satzstudio-hilger.de
Photos:	Mira Hampel Photography, www.mirahampel.de Adobe Stock: pg. 43 Paidotribo: pg. 31 top and bottom
Illustrations:	Pg. 33, Tensegrity model from Slomka, G.: Fasciae in Motion (4th edition), pg. 84 Adobe Stock, pg. 50
Managing editor:	Elizabeth Evans
Copyeditor:	Anne Rumery
Translator:	AAA Translations, St. Louis, MO

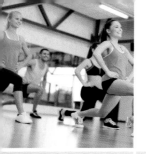

MORE GREAT FITNESS & HEALTH BOOKS

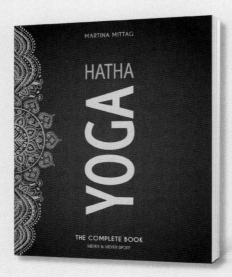

Martina Mittag

HATHA YOGA

The Complete Book

This is the most complete training book on hatha yoga. The various flows and progressions are suitable both for yoga instructors and practitioners. You will be introduced to yoga, including an overview of the origins and philosophy of classical yoga. This is followed by a detailed, practical section. The 34 best-known yoga asanas are presented, including their correct execution, symbolism, alignment, preparation, and guidance tips.

Specially coordinated series of exercises complete with photo progressions can be used for an hour session, either for a class or personal workouts. These series can be taken directly as they are or adapted to suit your needs. Also included are visualization and relaxation tips tailored to the photo progressions which all for a deeper immersion into the yoga practice.

424 p., in color
983 photos + illus.
Paperback, 8" x 10"
ISBN: 978-1-78255-185-0
$34.95 US

MEYER & MEYER Sport
Von-Coels-Str. 390
52080 Aachen
Germany

Phone +49 02 41 - 9 58 10 - 13
Fax +49 02 41 - 9 58 10 - 10
E-Mail sales@m-m-sports.com
Website www.thesportspublisher.com

All books available as E-books.

MEYER
& MEYER
SPORT

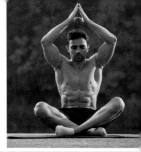

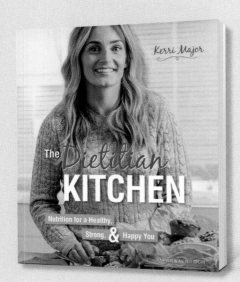

Kerri Major

THE DIETITIAN KITCHEN

Nutrition for a Healthy, Strong, & Happy You

As a registered dietitian and certified personal trainer, Kerri knows the importance of nourishing and fueling the body with a well-balanced diet and keeping active. However, the current diet trend, as often shared on social media, has caused people to develop a poor relationship with food—and their bodies.

This book brings you back to the basics of nutrition by encouraging everyone to learn the foundations of nutrition, providing the knowledge to nourish the body appropriately, and saying goodbye to fad diets for good! Its also provides more than 90 healthy, simple, affordable, and delicious recipes and exercise inspiration to help keep you moving. Kerri shares her nutrition and exercise philosophy and helps educate and inspire readers to look after themselves, showing them that it can be done, even with the busiest lifestyle.

312 p., in color
120 photos + illus.
Paperback, 8" x 10"
ISBN: 978-1-78255-184-3
$22.95 US

All information subject to change © Adobe Stock

MEYER & MEYER Sport
Von-Coels-Str. 390
52080 Aachen
Germany

Phone   +49 02 41 - 9 58 10 - 13
Fax   +49 02 41 - 9 58 10 - 10
E-Mail   sales@m-m-sports.com
Website   www.thesportspublisher.com

All books available as E-books.

MEYER
& MEYER
SPORT

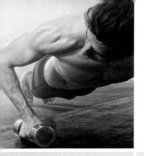

CHECK OUT OUR GREAT BOOKS

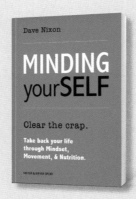

150 p., b/w
10 illus.
Paperback, 5.5" x 8.5"
ISBN: 978-1-78255-188-1
$14.95 US

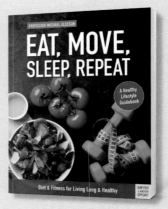

400 p., b/w
approx. 40 photos + illus.
Paperback, 7" x 10"
ISBN: 978-1-78255-187-4
$24.95 US

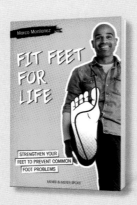

264 p., b/w
205 photos + illus.
Paperback, 5.5" x 8.5"
ISBN: 978-1-78255-183-6
$14.95 US

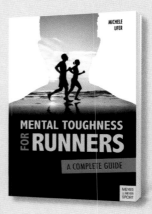

280 p., b/w
46 photos + illus.
Paperback, 5.5" x 8.5"
ISBN: 978-1-78255-161-4
$19.95 US

MEYER & MEYER SPORT

MEYER & MEYER Sport
Von-Coels-Str. 390
52080 Aachen
Germany

Phone   +49 02 41 - 9 58 10 - 13
Fax   +49 02 41 - 9 58 10 - 10
E-Mail   sales@m-m-sports.com
Website   www.thesportspublisher.com

All books available as E-books.

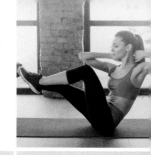

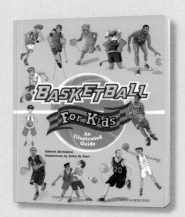

88 p., in color
approx. 200 illus.
Paperback, 9" x 11"
ISBN: 978-1-78255-173-7
$16.95 US

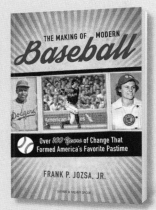

280 p., b/w
Paperback, 6" x 9"
ISBN: 978-1-78255-189-8

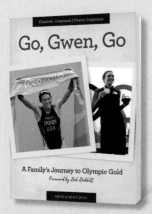

312 p., b/w
34 photos, in color
6" x 9"
ISBN: 978-1-78255-191-1
$24.95 US

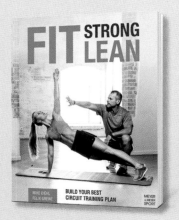

280 p., in color
395 photos + illus.
Paperback, 7" x 10"
ISBN: 978-1-78255-171-3
$19.95 US

All information subject to change © Adobe Stock

MEYER & MEYER Sport
Von-Coels-Str. 390
52080 Aachen
Germany

Phone   +49 02 41 - 9 58 10 - 13
Fax   +49 02 41 - 9 58 10 - 10
E-Mail   sales@m-m-sports.com
Website www.thesportspublisher.com

All books available as E-books.

MEYER
& MEYER
SPORT